INSIDE
IS
OUTSIDE

How stomach acid plays an essential role in Leaky Gut and why the Gastro-Test® is the missing link in diagnosing and treating the root causes of a host of seemingly unrelated symptoms from chronic fatigue and pain to eczema and depression.

by Dr. Tim McCullough
DC, DABCI, APC

Publishing Services provided by Paper Raven Books, LLC

Printed in the United States of America

First Printing, 2022

Paperback ISBN= 978-1-7376896-0-7

Hardback ISBN= 978-1-7376896-1-4

DISCLAIMER:
The information, including but not limited to, text, graphics, images and other material contained in this book are for informational purposes only. No material is intended to be a substitute for professional medical advice, diagnosis, or treatment. Always seek the advice of your physician or another qualified healthcare provider with any questions you may have regarding a medical condition or treatment and before undertaking a new health care regimen.

Table of Contents

Introduction

Why do I feel sick and fatigued all the time even though the doctors tell me there is nothing wrong?

Throughout my career as a functional medicine doctor treating thousands of chronically ill patients, I have seen nearly every symptom you can imagine, ranging from chronic fatigue and pain to skin diseases and serious neurological conditions, such as seizures and multiple sclerosis. These patients have often been told by medical providers when testing doesn't indicate a specific disease that it's all in their head or they're just depressed.

Even though these diverse symptoms may seem unrelated, they all have one fundamental thing in common: dysfunction of the body. A critical part of healing and health is learning that sickness is not some mystical entity; rather, it's a breakdown of normal body function. You don't have to be diagnosed with a disease to be sick. Most sickness begins with dysfunction of a normal body process and then progresses to a disease. When dysfunction is corrected, the illness and symptoms go away and health returns to normal. Of all the dysfunctions that can occur with chronic illness, Leaky Gut is almost always a major component.

This book teaches a key concept I have used daily to educate thousands of patients over the past 30 years about why they are functionally ill (meaning they are just able to function but are unable to perform normal activities without fatigue or pain). I wrote this book so that anyone, regardless of their background or prior knowledge, can understand and take steps towards treating the primary cause of many degenerative health conditions and diseases, which leave people feeling like something just isn't right and is typically accompanied by long-term chronic fatigue. I call the concept *"inside is outside."*

Most of us are probably familiar with the old adage: "You are what you eat." This is not true. In reality, you are what your intestinal wall allows into your body and what the intestines keep in to expel as waste. What is important to understand is that our bodies have developed a necessary and fine-tuned system to sort through what we take in from the outside world (like food and liquids) and to filter out the bad stuff and keep the good stuff.

This is the function of the digestive system, which is essentially a tube with a hole in the middle of it that runs the entire length of the body from where food and substances enter to where they leave (from the mouth to the anus). Nothing inside that tube should ever go beyond the digestive system boundaries (i.e., the intestinal wall) that the body doesn't specifically select and escort across the wall of the tube. In other words, the entire pathway from where food enters to where it leaves is actually still "outside" the body. The intestines must process and filter foods before crossing the intestinal wall and entering the "inside" of our body. This process is the key to health. When this system goes awry and chemicals and substances that should remain outside are allowed inside, dysfunction follows, leading to sickness and then disease. This is Leaky Gut in a nutshell.

Most chronic conditions and recovery depend on how well this very complex system works. Instead of "you are what you eat," a more accurate maxim would be: "You are what your digestive system determines you to be" (admittedly, this doesn't roll off the tongue quite as easily).

Throughout this book, we will explore how the digestive system works and how Leaky Gut develops when there is dysfunction in that system. You will learn that Leaky Gut is often the cause of chronic illness and how simple yet effective treatments can repair Leaky Gut and restore health. I also share real stories from patients whose health—and lives—have been transformed by this "inside is outside" approach. I hope to provide an accessible guide for understanding and treating Leaky Gut so that anyone who has been suffering from functional or chronic illness, or who is caring for a functionally or chronically ill loved one, has the knowledge and tools to finally find answers and start healing.

The word "doctor" comes from the Latin word for "teacher." I hope I can be just that for you with this book.

Dr. Tim McCullough; BS, M.Ed., DC, DABCI, APC

Foreword

Compiled on June 25, 2015 by Mikelle Challenger, mother of James Challenger, along with other medical and school documents pertaining to this summary. I give my permission for Dr. Tim McCullough to use any of the information to share with others.

James Challenger was born June 2007 at 38 weeks' gestation. 6 lbs. 1 oz. It was summer of 2014 that we began to see Dr. McCullough initially for James' severe eczema on his face (around his mouth) and arms. James also struggled with seizures and behavior, but we hoped to simply clear up the eczema, as that seemed more doable.

Dr. McCullough gave him ointment and oral drops. The eczema cleared up within days. After a few weeks, I noticed that when I stopped using the ointment it would come back. I asked Dr. McCullough and he said James needed a diet change to permanently stop the eczema. He also felt that James had a metal problem.

He had James evaluated and a hair biopsy done by August 2014. The results were stunning. James' copper levels were off the chart high and his lithium levels were non-existent. Dr. McCullough immediately began to treat both issues. We saw a huge difference in James' behavior and seizures. James was smiling and laughing, able to cope better. I was able to put him in a first grade class at church with the "regular" kids, and he was the only one to complete his book-memorizing scriptures. He was asked to sing a solo for the Christmas program and said a scripture on the mic and sang with the choir at the end-of-the-year program. We cried through it all.

Overall, his seizures have decreased to a point that we almost forget he has a problem. His seizures are less violent many times, only clonic. James has caught up at school and surpassed his own peers with song and scripture memorization at church. James is able to sit in a chair and concentrate while needing moderate redirection. He is socially able to play safely and happily with other children on playground sets and in swimming pools, two areas that were of great concern for me in the past. James (now 8) and Grant (now 5 ½) are the best of friends, though they do battle it out many afternoons.

James is a happy child who smiles, laughs, sings, plays, talks, and has friendly conversations with people. He is better now than we have ever known him. Dr. McCullough has given us back our son better than we ever have known him. James still has a long way to go, but we are for the very first time hopeful for James' future.

Mikelle Challenger, RN

CHAPTER 1

There Is Always an Answer

How conventional medicine has failed those suffering with chronic illness, and why your journey to health starts with functional medicine

Late one Friday afternoon at about 5:30 p.m. (it always happens that way on Fridays), a mom called and said her high school–aged daughter was in serious pain but was too embarrassed to come to the clinic with anyone there. I told the mom to come in after the last patient that day.

When this young lady walked in, I immediately understood what was causing her pain and embarrassment. Her lips were huge, black, cracked, and bleeding. She cringed in horrible pain whenever she tried to speak. Moreover, her emotional state was a wreck since she was supposed to be presented as the homecoming queen the next week.

This looked like a herpes infection, so I took her to an exam room and ran several tests to determine what medicine would help. Vitex herb was the herbal medicine the tests indicated was appropriate. Vitex is not known to be effective for a viral infection, but my experience has shown to go with the test results. So, I told the staff to mix up a salve with Vitex. I remember standing at the checkout counter with the mom and the patient and instructing the patient to take some of the salve and carefully rub it on her lips.

She gingerly applied the Vitex salve to her lips and rubbed it in as we all watched. Within a minute, she started to smile and said, "The pain is gone!" Then she started crying. You could see the hope in her eyes. I told her to keep applying the salve as necessary to keep the lips moist. She and her mom left, both clearly feeling relieved. On Monday morning, they came by the clinic for their follow-up appointment. Her lips were back to normal with just a bit of puffiness and redness. She was heading back to school, ready for her big night as the high school's newly crowned homecoming queen.

Even though the herb Vitex is not known for treating viral infections or for use on the skin, Vitex cream has become our go-to treatment for herpes. We continued our experiments and even came up with a variety of formulas, such as comfrey root mix for hemorrhoids and other combinations for general irritations of the skin. Hundreds of patients have benefitted from Vitex's effectiveness since the day that high school student was helped 25 years ago.

THINKING OUTSIDE THE BOX

There are physicians all around the world who are observing and questioning the effectiveness of treatments they were taught in school. They watch in futility as these treatments fail time after time. Many of us say to ourselves that we didn't go to school for 10 years (or more) and study every day for decades to watch failure after failure. So, we start experimenting with ideas we have and see how they work.

I have done these kinds of experiments in my practice for the past 30 years with a couple of important rules. First, do no harm. There would be no experimenting with anything that could potentially bring harm to the patient. Second, I would talk with the patient and tell them what I had in mind and what I expected to happen, and we would only move forward with the treatment if they understood and agreed. Third, we would give the treatment a reasonable amount of time to do its job and redo the test to see if it had worked.

For the past three decades, I have used this approach of trying things and discarding them if they didn't work, and keeping them and improving them if they did. Over the years, I have "discovered" amazing treatments that I have never read about or been taught but that are very effective with no risks or harmful side effects, like using Vitex salve for skin.

One of my goals in writing this book is to help you learn how to find doctors who think like this, because out-of-the-box thinking is often necessary to find real, lasting solutions for chronic illness.

DISEASE VS. HEALTH

What does it mean to be chronically ill or functionally ill? Functionally ill means that you are able to function in life but not well. You struggle to get through the day, feeling very fatigued, foggy-headed, in pain, or all of the above. You are functioning in your life but not at your normal capacity. Chronically ill means that you have a specific problem that you cannot seem to solve. This includes problems like migraine headaches, chronic pain, nausea, indigestion, rashes that won't resolve, and hot flashes. It also includes a diagnosed disease that allows you to live but makes you sick all the time, such as autoimmune diseases like lupus or Hashimoto's thyroid disease. Chronically or functionally ill does not mean you have a disease. More often than not, there is no disease, but there is dysfunction.

There are two primary approaches to medicine, and it is important to understand how the differences in their goals have a direct impact on treating chronic illness. In allopathic medicine (the more conventional, standard model), *disease* is the entity. In order to be treated within this framework, you must be diagnosed with a disease or condition. Otherwise, there is no treatment. In functional medicine, *health* is the entity. There often is not a primary disease present. The body is simply not functioning normally, and symptoms reflect the physical process(es) that has been disrupted and require treatment to return to normal.

Let's take chronic fatigue as an example. Standard (allopathic) doctors consider chronic fatigue an entity in and of itself, while functional (non-allopathic) doctors view chronic fatigue as a symptom resulting from physiological dysfunction. Some folks are chronically fatigued because they had a disease that was treated and their body is still not repaired from the trauma of the treatment and disease. We see this after surgery. The patient never returns to their previous health status because nothing was done to help the body to return to its previous levels of normal function.

Allopathic medicine has no answers for the functionally and chronically ill other than suppression of symptoms with drugs and surgery, which only offer temporary solutions that fail to address the root cause. In complex cases, such as chronic fatigue, a doctor with specialized training in physiological and functional medicine has real solutions because they are asking fundamentally different questions. They think in a different paradigm.

3

Allopathic medicine is important in emergencies, surgeries, and life-threatening problems where the body's natural functions or defenses are overwhelmed; in other words, it is the right approach in cases where a person has experienced serious damage or disruption beyond the body's ability to adapt to the trauma, and intervention is needed. This is what allopathic medicine is best at: outside intervention in life-threatening situations. These powerful treatments, including toxic medications and surgical procedures, are necessary because the threat is so severe that it takes overwhelming outside force to help the body deal with the damage. If you have headaches and there is an arrow stuck in your head, the first step is to remove the arrow. The allopathic doctor is very good at taking out arrows using drugs and surgery. Allopathic treatments might be necessary to save your life, but they do not create health. Remember, health is the goal of functional medicine.

Each kind of medicine has its place in health care, and this book will help teach you how and when to use each one.

JOURNEY TO HEALTH

One common trend I see in my patients with chronic illness is that they start to question themselves. *What did I do that caused this? The doctors can't find anything, so am I really sick or is it my imagination? Maybe I'm just depressed?* This kind of thinking contributes to a vicious cycle of emotional trauma, which is compounded by the fear of the unknown. It is critical to be evaluated and tested for fatal or genetic conditions, such as cancer or dementia; if this fear is not put to bed with testing and facts, it may destroy your hope of getting well.

Once you decide to get well and commit to finding answers, your life-long journey of healing can begin. It starts with the decision to take personal responsibility for yourself and solidify your determination to become healthy. You must make up your mind to do whatever you have to do to survive and thrive. You must make a commitment to find the professionals who can help you, doctors who think outside of the box. You must accept that you will have to do things that are not in line with traditional medical testing and treatment.

As a chronically ill patient who most likely doesn't have medical training, searching for help can become a hardship all on its own. It will be difficult and filled with temporary failures. Keep in mind that failure is an important part of success; limiting the failures to small ones, financially and emotionally, is the goal. You have to remind yourself after each failure that *there is always an answer, I just haven't found it yet*. You must find doctors who believe that too.

Doctors are not trained that way. Most are fatalists, viewing their patients' fates as more or less predetermined by the disease they have. They are trained to fit you in a box (disease), and if that box isn't in their area of expertise, then it is out of their hands. You have to learn what kind of doctor can and will have the attitude of hope, a doctor who believes they will find an answer. If I learn of something new that might help a patient I saw years before, I call them and tell them I found something that might help them. Often, that new piece of information makes a big difference or even completely solves their problem. I never stop searching for answers to help my patients; that is the kind of doctor you need.

Make a commitment to yourself that you will continue to search until you find what you need. You will have to learn a lot and can leave no stone unturned. You will have to adapt to maneuvering your way around every aspect of allopathic, osteopathic, chiropractic, and alternative medicine. It may be tempting to turn to Dr. Internet, but please do so with caution as there is a lot of incorrect information out there. To be honest, most doctors who know what they are doing in functional medicine wouldn't post their work on the internet because it puts them at risk with the medical, chiropractic, and osteopathic boards that are not friendly to doctors who use natural treatments, no matter how scientific or effective they are. You will have to find the great doctors by doing some digging, word-of-mouth, and person-to-person communications. Remember, *a great physician needs no trumpet*.

I wrote this book to help you find answers and guidance in your journey to health. In over 30 years of practice and thousands of cases, I have found time and time again that the first place to look for trouble is in the stomach, especially the level of hydrochloric acid, which is one of the primary mechanisms of Leaky Gut. Even though it is one of the keys to health, it is often totally ignored. In the next chapter, we'll explore why stomach acid is a critical piece of the chronic illness puzzle.

CHAPTER 2

Anything Can Cause Anything

How multiple symptoms can have one cause, and why Leaky Gut is often at the center of seemingly unrelated chronic illness experiences

Sherry was 10 years old when she came to see me. She was a talented gymnast and was top ranked in the state, but recently she had developed severe pain in her knees and ankles that prevented her from being able to practice anymore. Her x-rays indicated that she had Osgood-Schlatter disease, where inflammation caused by repetitive intense physical activity results in a painful, bony bump near the bottom of the knee. The pain is caused by a tearing of the patella tendon from the bone at the insertion of the tendon. It's a condition that is commonly seen among young athletes and often ends their careers.

She saw her primary care physician, who recommended what most doctors do for this condition: stop athletics. Quite frankly, this is why coaches and athletes dislike doctors. In the athletes' and coaches' minds, this is not an option. Being an old athlete myself, I understand that, to these kids, sports is their life. They are looking for a "fix," not to be told to end what they love to do and stop being who they are. Fortunately, there are solutions for these kids other than being told to find something else to do with their lives.

Sherry also presented with severe eczema, which was not responding to treatment prescribed by her dermatologist. While eczema is not debilitating, it is a major clue for a functional medicine physician. I understood that the rash and the knee and ankle pain were related and part of the same cause of her problems. One of the things we do with eczema is test for food allergies. We started by testing for allergies with blood work. The results revealed an allergy to corn. Eliminating corn from her diet cleared up her eczema, and having even just a bite of corn would cause a flare-up, confirming that the eczema was related to the corn allergy.

We also treated her knees with ice therapy, stretching, and anti-inflammatory medication including non-steroidal anti-inflammatories and homeopathic medicines. The results were intermittent. When she had intense workouts, her knees would become inflamed, which would result in tendonitis. We were seeing small amounts of improvement with the elimination of corn from the diet and the other treatments, but clearly we had not found the root cause of the inflammation yet.

I spoke to Sherry's mom and shared my thoughts about testing for stomach acid levels. Normally, young kids like Sherry do not have serious stomach acid level problems, but because of her eczema and limited response to the treatment, I believed there may be a core issue with the digestive system. I explained that if she was not digesting and absorbing proteins properly, it could cause both the tendonitis and the food allergies. I explained to Sherry that if she was not digesting proteins, her tendons would not repair and they would be inflamed because they are made of protein. Mom agreed to testing, and we performed the Gastro-Test®, Indican test, and pancreatic enzyme test (we will explore these tests more in Chapter 7).

The results showed that she was making stomach acid but not enough when she was eating protein. Sherry started by taking one hydrochloric acid (HCl) and pepsin tablet per meal and increased the dose every two days. When she reached seven pills per day, all of the pain and inflammation in her knees and joints disappeared and her eczema cleared up, even if she ate corn. If she dropped to six capsules, the symptoms reappeared. Once she found her optimal dose, she was able to return to her gymnastics training.

As her body started to correct itself with properly digested and absorbed protein, she was able to reduce the HCl dose over time and work towards not needing it at all eventually. Identifying the problem early in life undoubtedly saved this young lady from a lot of heartache and sickness in the future and allowed her to continue pursuing her passion for gymnastics.

Patients often ask me how they know if what we are doing is working. It is really simple. Do you get better? Have the symptoms you were having reduced or gone to zero? If you are not taking drugs to eliminate the symptoms and the symptoms disappear with the treatment, it means two things: the diagnosis is right and the treatment is effective. When the body stops producing the pain or symptoms and no drugs have been used to cover them up, then you know the body is healing itself. This is true healing that produces health.

***

Trina was a 58-year-old woman who had been experiencing debilitating fatigue among a host of other symptoms, including bloating, constipation, menopausal symptoms, mid-back and neck pain, and thinning hair. She was understandably miserable and was at the point where she just wasn't able to function anymore because of the severe fatigue. She, like so many other patients who have walked through my doors, was one of "the functionally ill"; they have the minimum amount of functionality to get through each day but feel horrible and barely have enough energy to live life. It is a horrible way to live.

Trina's physical exam and extensive blood work revealed nothing unusual. Aside from being pale, slightly overweight, and having some puffiness around the eyes, she looked "normal." She had previously been prescribed thyroid medication and had seen a nutritionist and acupuncturist. Nothing had helped. After running our normal battery of tests, we did the Gastro-Test®, Indican test, and pancreatic enzyme test. The results indicated severe hypochlorhydria (i.e., low levels of stomach acid) and low pancreatic enzyme production, which meant that her body was not able to break down food sufficiently. We started with a simple treatment that included large doses of HCl prior to meals and pancreatic enzymes after meals.

At our three-week follow-up, Trina reported staggering improvement. Her fatigue had improved by 80%, bloating and gas by 60%, neck and mid-back pain by 50%, and her constipation, hot flashes, and sleep problems had completely resolved. At our six-week follow-up, her pain had also completely resolved, and her fatigue and gastrointestinal symptoms were almost entirely gone. At week six, we started her on vitamin and nutrient therapy to start her rebuilding process. She would have to stay on the HCl therapy long-term, since we don't heal as quickly and generally produce less HCl as we age. But after years of suffering, Trina finally had her life back once we addressed the root cause of her issues.

MULTIPLE SYMPTOMS, ONE CAUSE

What did Sherry and Trina have in common? On the surface, their cases seem vastly different. Sherry was a young athlete sidelined by severe pain in her knees and ankles due to inflammation and tendonitis, and Trina was in her 50s and was battling a host of chronic ailments, including debilitating fatigue. While their symptoms were completely different, they could all be traced back to one source: Leaky Gut due to lack of HCl production or low stomach acid.

Their cases demonstrate a critical concept: any one disease or condition can have multiple causes and any one cause can result in multiple symptoms. In the words of chiropractic icon Dr. William Harper, "anything can cause anything." The idea that one "thing" causes a disease or that one group of strictly defined symptoms maps onto a disease is a rather simplistic view given the complexity of how the body functions. The field of medicine would not have developed thousands of tests if this were the case. And tests are important; diagnostic testing combined with the doctor's thinking process are the key to diagnosis. Symptoms are not the key. I have patients who drive themselves crazy by spending hours on the internet looking at what symptom is associated with what disease. (Please don't do that. It's bad for your mental health.) We have known for years that it is not true that one bacteria, one virus, or one cause is responsible for symptoms, but it is an easy idea to sell to the public. Everyone would like to find the silver bullet to make all the problems go away. The body isn't that simple, and that approach is surely not the path to attain health.

Sherry and Trina illustrate this concept of "anything can cause anything." When there seemed to be no answer to their illnesses in allopathic medicine, an accurate functional diagnosis obtained with proper testing and a simple treatment centered on repairing, restoring, and healing their Leaky Gut allowed them to return to normal life.

MULTIPLE SYMPTOMS ONE CAUSE

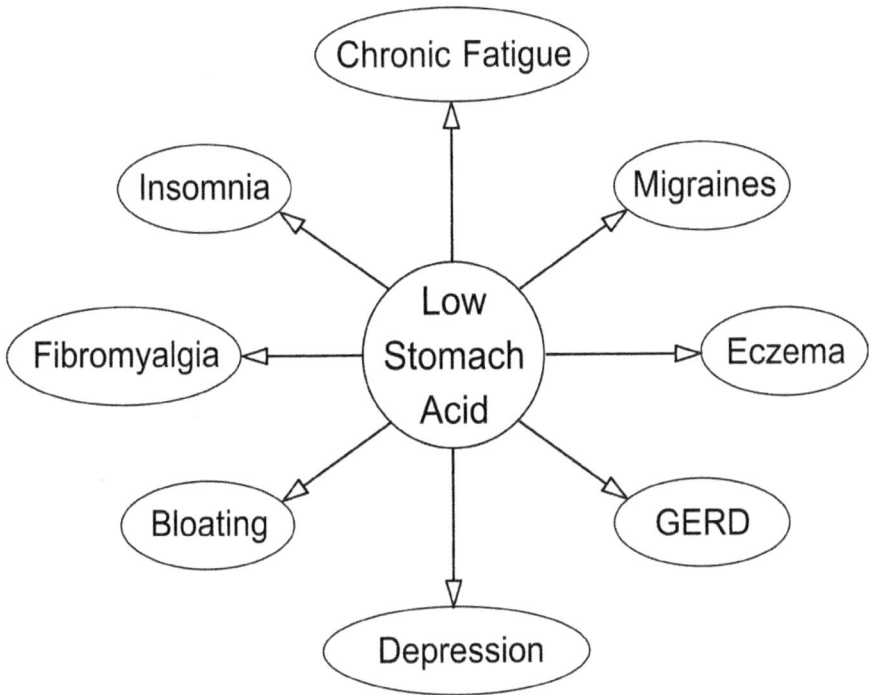

CHAPTER 3

Basics of the Digestive System

How the digestive system works, and why its function (and dysfunction) is the key to health (and chronic illness)

To truly understand what Leaky Gut is and why it is almost always an essential driver of functional and chronic illness, we need to first understand how the digestive system works when everything is operating as it should be. Remember: illness is a result of dysfunction, and restoring health depends on the body being able to function normally.

THE MOUTH: CHEWING AND SWALLOWING

The beginning of the digestive system is the oral cavity of the mouth and the end is the anus. These are the gates that control what goes in and what goes out. The intestinal tract is essentially one long tube that acts like a tunnel carrying substances and chemicals through your body. This tunnel, which runs from the mouth to the anus, is called the *lumen*. We'll return to this important concept soon.

First, let's start at the beginning of the digestive process: the mouth. Food or liquid entering the mouth is initially unknown to your body. Whether you've just put a sip of coffee, a fresh vegetable, or a sugary treat into your mouth, your body doesn't know what it is until the food has been analyzed and each chemical has been identified by the nervous system. This gears up the rest of the digestive system so that it can be ready to process the new substance. Taste buds are the key players here. As sensory and neurological receptors, their role is to analyze the chemical make-up of the food or liquid and to signal the body to start manufacturing digestive enzymes. These enzymes are specific types of proteins that help break down food. Our bodies have thousands of such chemicals, which are necessary to "actively transport" the good stuff to the parts of the body where it is needed and to discharge what is not needed. Taste buds are the neurological workhorses that do the heavy lifting of chemical analysis.

When you are eating foods (as opposed to drinking liquids), chewing plays an important part in this process. Chewing is primarily under voluntary control, meaning you can choose to chew food as much or as little as you want, but the rest of the digestive process is primarily under automatic or *autonomic* control of the nervous system. This autonomic system controls the production of saliva by three pairs of salivary glands that lubricate, clean, and moisten as well as capture dangerous chemicals to be processed out of the body such as mercury and lead. Our bodies create about two quarts, or eight cups, of saliva every day.

Chewing is more important than we usually realize, not only because it breaks down the food into smaller particles for swallowing but also because it "cracks" open the food and allows the individual chemical components to be released. Then the taste buds analyze them and send the information to the digestive system through the nervous system, which starts the process of manufacturing digestive enzymes and other chemicals that the body will need to digest and absorb the food that's being chewed. In fact, studies have shown that rats that don't chew their food are less healthy than those that do, and sick rats that are allowed to chew can return to good health. By providing a chemical analysis of food and kicking systems into gear, taste buds and chewing both play key roles in digestion.

If you've already done some research around the digestive system or somehow retained what you learned in high school biology, you may remember that chewing stimulates the manufacture of certain proteins, releasing hydrochloric acid, pepsin, pancreatic enzymes, and the thousands of transporter molecules in the small and large intestines needed to transport the selected substances and nutrients into the body through the intestinal wall. This includes the essential amino acids and fatty acids that are necessary for life.

Once you have chewed and thoroughly mixed the food with enzymes, you swallow, and the food enters the esophagus. The esophagus is a

10-inch muscular tube that transports the chewed food from the mouth to the stomach. The lining of the mouth and esophagus are made up of "squamous cells," which means they are smooth, wet, and slippery, and they are very sensitive to chemicals.

There is a valve between the stomach and the esophagus called the lower esophageal sphincter that acts as a secure gateway. Once the food is inside the stomach, the valve closes very tightly and prevents the stomach contents from refluxing and damaging the delicate lining of the esophagus. It is critical that the contents of the stomach do not "reflux" back into the esophagus because it is very painful and can cause diseases. The valve should remain closed at all times except when food or liquid is passing from the esophagus down to the stomach. This valve can become damaged with chronic reflux, and surgery to repair damaged valves has had questionable success rates in my experience.

Once the food is in the stomach, certain types of cells start to make hydrochloric acid and gastrin (a hormone that produces gastric juice), both of which are used to break down the food and kill off any substances or critters that shouldn't be there, like viruses and chemicals. The stomach muscles start mixing the food together with the acids and juices, preparing it for the next phase of digestion in the small intestine, where the real work begins. The stomach is a mixing tank, and its role to the digestive process is critical and depends on having appropriate amounts of acid.

The contents of the stomach are then released through the pyloric sphincter into the small intestines. Just like the lower esophageal sphincter, it is a secure gateway that remains tightly closed until conditions signal that it is time to open up and allow substances to pass from one area of digestion to the next. This pyloric sphincter requires the mixture to have specific acidic levels in order to open and move the contents from the stomach to the small intestine. If the contents of the stomach are not prepared enough (meaning the hydrochloric acid levels are too low), then they remain in the stomach and continue to be mixed and broken down until they are ready to move to the small intestine.

The muscles of the small intestine then mix with digestive juices from the pancreas, liver, and intestine, further breaking down the food and absorbing water and digested nutrients into the bloodstream. This absorption in the small intestines is the key to health and is accomplished primarily through active transport (an important process that we will explore more in Chapter 5). Whatever is not absorbed in the small intestine moves on to the large intestine, which includes the colon, rectum, and anus. The large intestine continues absorbing nutrients and water and then converts undigested waste into solid matter. This remaining material then exits the body through the anus in the form of feces.

That, in a nutshell, is the digestive process in a well-functioning system.

LUMEN: THE OUTSIDE WORLD INSIDE

The entire tunnel from your mouth through the stomach, small intestines, and large intestines is the *lumen*. This is essentially a hole through the middle of your body and thus technically is still outside of your body. The wall of the lumen is a protective and selective barrier that exists to either transport food and substances into the body or stop them from entering the body. This protective wall of the lumen allows the body to transport chemicals, proteins, fats, and nutrients from food across the intestinal wall—the sides of the tunnel—and then discard the unwanted chemicals and waste products out through the anus in the form of feces.

If food particles, viruses, bacteria, fungi, parasites, or chemicals that enter the mouth and proceed into the lumen cross the barrier without being escorted by specialized transporters through the wall of the intestines, then the body reacts to these materials as an invader. These unescorted substances that get into the body are called *antigens*. The immune system identifies them as problems and attempts to remove them.

The body does not like things it hasn't selected for use inside of itself. The nervous system perceives them as threats to life. Substances that breach the barrier are declared the enemy. Even undigested food that is not properly escorted across this barrier by the correct transporter system will become your enemy. The body's immune system activates to defend you against these antigens and increases the battle's intensity to whatever level is necessary to keep you alive. The first indication that a battle is underway is a symptom of some sort. While this could be many different symptoms, the most common ones are headaches, eczema, skin issues, swelling, and fatigue.

Leaky Gut is the condition that results from your body's immune system going to war with the enemy (antigens) that breached the barrier. Bacteria, viruses, parasites, pollen, dust, dirt, insects, and numerous chemicals, such as mercury and nickel, enter your digestive system on a daily basis. Mucus does its job in the nose and mouth by trapping all the dirt, pollen, and critters, and whatever goes on to be swallowed then moves on to your stomach, which will kill or destroy all of the remaining invaders. However, this requires having a functioning *stomach acid barrier,* which requires a proper hydrochloric acid level in the stomach. Without an appropriately functioning stomach acid barrier, enemies leak across what should be a protected wall that separates the "outside" world from the "inside" of the body, leading the immune system to launch into a guided attack mode that results in a vast range of symptoms. Stomach acid levels are at the core of this process.

CHAPTER 4

Stomach Acid Barrier

How the stomach acid barrier enables the digestive system to function, and why hydrochloric acid is the key to identifying and resolving Leaky Gut

The stomach acid barrier is one of the most important systems in the body and is critical to health, yet it is mostly ignored in orthodox medicine. Its key player, hydrochloric acid (HCl), performs a number of essential functions in your digestive system:

1. Forms the stomach acid barrier.

2. Kills bacteria, viruses, parasites, and fungi.

3. Mixes food and prepares protein for absorption in the small intestines.

4. Renders calcium and iron salts suitable for digestion, which maintains bone health and prevents osteoporosis.

5. Helps make intrinsic factor, a chemical that is critical for the absorption of essential nutrients, such as B12 and folic acid, which prevent neurological disease.

If there is not enough acid in the stomach even when it is empty, antigens including bacteria and viruses can pass through the stomach without being destroyed and are allowed to enter the small intestines. Once there, they can be absorbed into the body, causing infections or chronic illnesses such as migraine headaches, chronic fatigue, insomnia, autoimmune disorders, and skin conditions. When the body is fighting antigens—whether they are bacteria, viruses, or undigested food particles—day after day, month after month, and year after year, this constant war by the immune system results in a host of chronic conditions including fatigue. This is Leaky Gut. With a properly functioning stomach acid barrier, HCl kills and destroys bacteria and viruses quickly before this scenario can happen.

There are very few drugs for this condition. There are no adrenal-boosting supplements or magic vitamins or exotic foods from some far-off land to cure this situation. The cure is to identify and prevent these antigens from crossing the normal barrier of the digestive system and to heal the gut lining so the gastrointestinal transport system works properly. When the body is no longer a war zone and the immune system does not have to fight an onslaught of antigens after each meal or after each swallow, the symptoms resolve and health returns.

The reason allopathic medicine is typically unable to help chronic conditions is because doctors in this paradigm are trained to diagnose and treat the damage after the body breaks down and has developed symptoms that can be categorized and labelled a disease. If there is no diagnosable disease or damage to repair or treat, then orthodox medicine's treatment is "palliative." In other words, prescribe medications to relieve the symptoms. In fact, almost every treatment for non-diseased gastrointestinal tract is a form of acid reduction therapy. You see this in medicines such as antacids, acid blockers, and calcium products that are all designed to reduce acid. These therapies may reduce symptoms temporarily, but they do not address the root cause and, in fact, can exacerbate dysfunction.

One of the greatest myths in medicine is that too much acid causes gastrointestinal problems. What I have discovered in 30 years of practice with chronic illness and the latest gastrointestinal research is the very opposite: the lack of acid results in Leaky Gut and is the root problem that causes a host of seemingly unrelated symptoms. For anyone who has been suffering and has been unable to find answers, this is very likely the missing piece of their body's ability to completely heal itself. Measuring the production of stomach's acid production is the place to start with any chronic health condition.

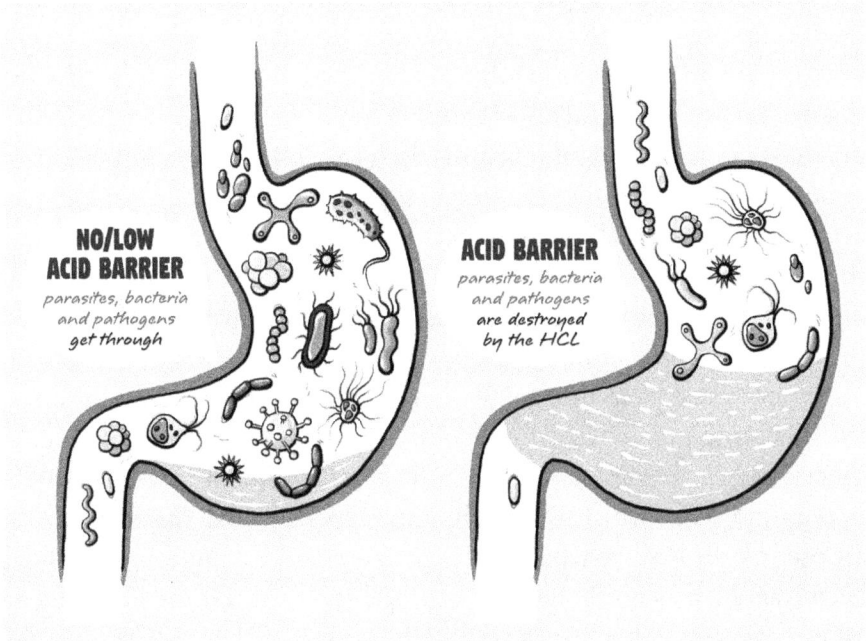

NO/LOW ACID BARRIER
parasites, bacteria and pathogens get through

ACID BARRIER
parasites, bacteria and pathogens are destroyed by the HCL

ACID REFLUX

For almost a century, doctors and scientists believed that ulcers were caused by too much acid. The fact is that ulcers are caused by a bacterium called *H. pylori*. Yet another and more damaging myth continues. Most people think, and orthodox medicine still tells patients, that too much acid in the stomach is the cause of reflux or any number of uncomfortable symptoms. Actually, HCl is absolutely essential in the gastrointestinal system and we now know too little acid is the reason why most folks have reflux.

Reflux occurs when undigested contents of the stomach go back up through the valve into the esophagus instead of being moved along down to the small intestines. This is very painful because the esophagus is not able to tolerate even a small amount of acid. It is lined with squamous cell tissue, which is smooth and soft like the mouth, and acid destroys the tissue. Reflux can also cause chest and back pain due to the muscles in the esophagus spasming. The short-term answer is to neutralize the acid in the esophagus with a base like baking soda. But, over the long term, especially with acid-suppressing drugs, this makes the problem worse.

Recent studies in gastroenterology have shown that low hydrochloric levels cause the two valves—the lower esophageal sphincter at the top of the stomach and the pyloric sphincter at the bottom of the stomach—to not work normally. These valves are critical to understanding why a person develops gastroesophageal reflux disease (GERD) or reflux. As you may remember from the earlier chapter on the digestive system, the sphincters act as gateways that allow substances to pass from one area of digestion to the next (from the esophagus to the stomach to the small intestines). These gateways need to be opened at very specific times, and if anything interferes with this timing, problems ensue.

Stomach acid levels determine when the valve from the stomach and to the small intestines open primarily by breaking down protein in food. If there is sufficient stomach acid, then the proteins in food are broken down into amino acids, which are the building blocks of life. These molecules are used by the body to repair tissue, grow cells, and manufacture essential chemicals such as hormones and neurotransmitters. Of the 20 different amino acids the body needs to function, nine of them are considered essential, meaning that the body cannot make them on its own and must get them through foods or supplements.

What is important to understand about this process is that proteins are broken down into amino acids in the stomach, our digestive system's mixing tank. The stomach requires a certain level of acid to break down protein sufficiently before it can pass on to the next phase of digestion in the small intestines. The valve from the stomach to the small intestines will not open until the substances are properly prepared. If acid levels are too low and the stomach is unable to break everything down in a timely manner, then the lower valve to the small intestines stays closed, forcing the food to stay in the stomach to continue to be mixed and prepared. As the stomach continues to squeeze and push contents in an effort to break everything down, the food gets pushed back up towards the esophagus, forcing the acidic mixture into the upper valve and causing pain and discomfort. This is reflux.

There are two other important processes related to stomach acid levels at this phase: (a) destroying unwanted guests such as viruses and chemicals and (b) breaking down protein into amino acids. We'll discuss these in more detail later, but just remember that these depend on the stomach having sufficient hydrochloric acid. If the stomach is unable to do either of these things properly, it sets the stage for serious problems in the small intestines, where the most important parts of digestion take place (i.e., absorbing and transporting nutrients and sorting what the body needs from waste products).

Why does the myth that reflux is caused by too much acid continue? It's simple: doctors do not test their patients' stomach acid levels. Think about it for a minute. If you spoke to everyone you know who has been told by a doctor they have reflux and asked them if the doctor tested their stomach acid levels prior to prescribing the drug, not a single person would say yes. As ridiculous as it sounds, testing is not part of the protocol. A doctor friend of mine asked one of his gastroenterologist colleagues why he doesn't test stomach acid, and he responded by saying, "It doesn't matter. I was trained in medical school to give acid blockers for reflux, and that is what I do."

If a mechanic told you that you have too much air in your tires, you would likely ask them how they know that. They would tell you that they used an air pressure gauge to measure the PSI and determine whether there was too much, too little, or just the right amount of air. But, for some reason, doctors aren't trained to do the same thing with something as important and as easily measurable as stomach acid. It doesn't matter if you have a $200,000 Mercedes in pristine condition; if the tires have gone flat because they don't have the right amount of air, that car isn't going anywhere. The digestive system is the same; without the right amount of stomach acid, it just isn't going to function properly.

Acid-blocking drugs can cause serious disease and side effects, including poor absorption of vitamins and minerals, asthma, allergies, skin diseases, lupus, rheumatoid arthritis, ulcerative colitis, and increased risk for certain types of cancer and infections. Prescribing these medications without proper testing is unacceptable. Patients should not be put on any acid-blocking drugs unless a test has been run to prove whether there is too much stomach acid. If you ever find yourself in this position, you can and should insist on having tests run and refuse treatment if your doctor is unwilling to do this. Demand from your doctor at least the same level of care as the mechanic gives your car.

PATIENT STORY: BACK PAIN AND STOMACH ACID

Lamar had suffered from intermittent back pain for years. One day, he came into my office and said his reflux was so bad he couldn't sleep or eat. When asked to describe where the pain was, he identified the area between his shoulders in the mid-back. His other doctor (of course) had put him on acid blockers, which (of course) were not working. I asked him if that doctor had done a test to measure stomach acid levels. He said no. I told him the only way to know what was going on was to test his stomach acid levels and explained that reflux in most cases is caused by too little stomach acid, not too much. We administered the Gastro-Test® and checked his pancreatic enzyme levels.

His tests indicated that he was hypochlorhydric, meaning his stomach acid levels were too low. I prescribed betaine HCl and pepsin along with pancreatic enzymes with meals. After a few weeks, the reflux stopped and never returned. His mid-back pain was relieved because the nerves from the stomach originate in the mid-back. When the irritation of the stomach nerves stopped, so did the pain. (We'll explore this concept of interconnected systems in Chapter 6.)

When he asked me why other doctors don't prescribe HCl, I told him they simply don't do the test. They fail to question the myth they learned in school that reflux is too much stomach acid instead of using science. Lamar is a happy man and sleeps well now.

HOW MUCH ACID IS NORMAL?

Normally, the average person's stomach produces almost half a gallon of hydrochloric acid each day. And if you eat foods with high amounts of protein, like meat and beans, you will produce even more. So, what causes low levels of stomach acid levels?

The major reasons why the stomach doesn't produce enough acid are (a) nutritional deficiencies due to malabsorption and (b) acid-suppressive drugs. When acid levels are low, minerals such as calcium, magnesium, and potassium and vitamins like B12 and folic acid, which are necessary for life, are not absorbed properly. This causes malabsorption syndrome, meaning the body lacks the necessary materials to make stomach acid and enzymes and to repair tissue. This problem is really critical in children like Sherry, the 10-year-old competitive gymnast who was sidelined due to knee and ankle pain that was caused by insufficient stomach acid levels. At those young ages, their bones, muscles, and nervous system—including the brain—are still developing. It is a well-known fact that children with malabsorption problems have a reduced life span and are prone to sickness in their adult life.

Calcium is essential for life, and so are many of the vitamins and nutrients that we are eating to make our bodies healthier. Even if you are *eating* the right foods, if your stomach and intestinal tract is not *breaking down* that food so that it can be *absorbed* and used by your body, you can become sick and functionally ill. Without adequate acid in the stomach, the entire digestive process breaks down. As we age, we naturally produce less stomach acid, and folks over the age of 50 are more likely to have low HCl levels and experience the accompanying negative health effects.

As one example of the importance of stomach acid's role in absorbing vital nutrients, several years ago a major drug manufacturer attempted to advertise their new antacid product made of calcium as osteoporosis prevention. The FDA forced them to remove the ad because, while it is true that calcium is essential for strong bones, stomach acid levels must be normal to absorb calcium and suppressing acid levels with an antacid interrupts the absorption.

On the other hand, too much HCl also presents a problem. In medicine, too much of anything is a cause for alarm. Even though estrogen and thyroid are essential hormones, too much estrogen is associated with breast cancer and too much thyroid hormone can pose a life-threatening situation. Excessive endocrine, or hormone, secretion in the body is generally a red flag for something bad, such as tumors, growths, and cancers. While most doctors would agree with this, for some reason too much acid is treated like it is normal. In my clinic where we test every patient for stomach acid, I rarely see levels that are too high. A test result that indicates high levels of HCl is a red flag, and we always dig deeper to figure out what is going on and how to treat it or refer to a specialist.

DISEASE PREVENTION

Another important function of HCl is disease prevention. When your body is exposed to viruses, bacteria, pollens, chemicals, or environmental irritants in the air, the mucus in your nose and respiratory system traps it. When you swallow this mucus, it cleans your airways from these potential pathogens or environmental insults. After they are swallowed and enter the digestive system, HCl destroys them in your stomach and prevents these pathogens from being absorbed into the bloodstream and infecting you through the intestinal wall. The stomach acid barrier is a major part of your body's protection against communicable diseases such as the flu and other viruses and bacteria.

Because the stomach acid barrier plays such a critical role in eliminating pathogens, absorbing nutrients, and preventing disease, it is essential to work with a doctor to measure whether your stomach acid barrier is present and whether your HCl levels are enough to protect you. When stomach acid levels are too low, the dysfunction in the digestive system leads to the gut becoming "leaky," which can result in a wide range of debilitating symptoms and chronic illness.

CHAPTER 5

Active Transport System

How Leaky Gut happens, and why the active transport system is at the heart of dispelling the myth that "you are what you eat"

In the previous chapters, we explored how the digestive system functions and why sufficient levels of hydrochloric acid (HCl) are essential to this process, dispelling the myth that many gastrointestinal issues, especially reflux, are caused by too much stomach acid. With the goal of you being an informed patient, I'm going to share a fairly detailed explanation of exactly what's happening inside your gastrointestinal tract when your gut becomes "leaky."

DYSBIOSIS: WHERE THE LEAKS START

Many serious, chronic problems occur because the biome of the intestinal tract is not functioning normally, a condition called *dysbiosis*. You can think of the biome as a home for important microorganisms that live inside your digestive tract, including bacteria, viruses, and fungi. In fact, there are about four pounds of these critters living inside each of us, and they help support a variety of important health functions, such as digesting certain foods, making essential vitamins and nutrients, and defending against harmful toxins and pathogens. When the biome is a happy home, this environment has the right amount of everything it needs, including acids, enzymes, and chemicals, and the types and amounts of critters are in balance. However, if certain things are missing or if there is an overgrowth of these microorganisms, then it becomes an unhappy home and the walls containing it start to fail, allowing contents from the biome to leak into your body. This is not good, especially when it occurs in the small intestines.

Let's think of the gut as a classroom full of children. If all the kids are doing their work and are minding the rules, then the classroom environment is functioning normally in a way that allows the students to learn. If several students are talking and causing disruption, the environment of that classroom becomes abnormal and the children have a more difficult time concentrating and learning. If a majority of the kids become unruly, then there is a breakdown of the entire system. In this situation, the classroom itself is normal: the desks are not broken, the lights work, etc. But the individual players are not doing what they are supposed to do, which is sit quietly and do their work without disturbing the other kids. The classroom is dysfunctional.

Your gut is similar in dysbiosis. The structure of the digestive system is okay (e.g., all the major parts are there and intact), but the bacteria and chemicals in the biome are out of balance. This causes a dysfunction of the digestive process because the walls of the intestines no longer act as a functioning barrier and Leaky Gut is the result.

The best way to fix this problem is to correct only the children who are not doing their work. If those few kids start behaving, then the classroom becomes functional. The same is true in the digestive tract. When you balance the levels of enzymes, chemicals, bacteria, and viruses, the biome returns to normal. Killing all the bacteria in the gut with antibiotics is not the answer in the same way that killing all the kids in the classroom would not be the answer. The goal is to create a happy home where everything is in balance and all the players are functioning in the way they are supposed to.

SMALL INTESTINES: THE GATEKEEPERS

As you may recall from earlier chapters, the small intestines play a critical role in absorbing nutrients by breaking food down into proteins, fats, and carbohydrates, chemical building blocks that are necessary for a variety of functions. This involves sorting what should be delivered throughout the body from what should continue to move through the digestive tract and be expelled. The small intestines are a muscular tube that measures about six and a half feet in length and sits between the stomach (where food is broken down) and large intestines (where waste is processed). The small intestines receive partially digested food from the stomach, a type of digestive fluid called bile from the liver and gallbladder, and a mixture of enzymes to break down sugars, fats, and starches from the pancreas. All of these elements work together to process food, absorb what the body needs through a finely tuned filtration and active transport system, and pass nutrients on to the bloodstream for delivery to other areas of the body.

The workhorse of the small intestines are the *microvilli*. These tiny hairlike structures form a specialized brush border throughout the small intestines where the "active transport" of nutrients, vitamins, and minerals take place. Active is the keyword here, because the process requires a large amount of energy and effort in order to ensure the right substances are escorted across the intestinal wall at the right time. This system must function properly to have a healthy gut. It is one of the fundamental systems of life. I cannot emphasize strongly enough how important this selective active transport system is to your health. ***The breakdown of the active transport system can result in a myriad of seemingly unrelated symptoms and is responsible or part of almost every chronic health problem.***

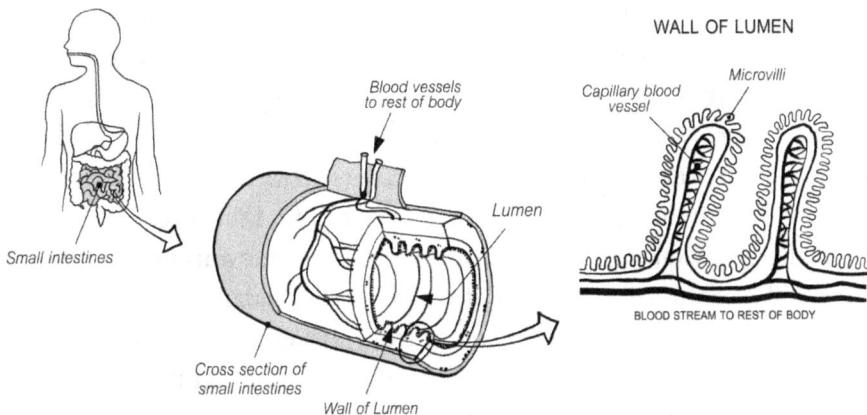

WALL OF LUMEN

Microvilli

Blood vessels to rest of body

Capillary blood vessel

Lumen

Small intestines

Cross section of small intestines

Wall of Lumen

BLOOD STREAM TO REST OF BODY

WARNING SIGNS

Remember how we talked about the lumen of the intestinal tract really being outside your body? Food goes in the mouth and waste products come out at the rectum. The tube inside the digestive tract—the lumen—is "outside" the body and all substances should stay there unless they are selected and escorted across the intestinal wall by the body itself. When this barrier is breached in the small intestines and the active transport system fails, problems of disease and sickness from dysbiosis and Leaky Gut begin. One of the primary symptoms is fatigue, though there are a multitude of symptoms that can occur.

Some of the first symptoms of initial digestive trouble are gas, belching, swelling of the stomach and abdomen, constipation, diarrhea, and reflux. These symptoms are telling your body that the digestive tract is not working well and is going to break down if it isn't corrected. Do not just ignore these first symptoms or take medication like acid blockers and antacids to cover them up. These are your body's warning signs telling you that something is wrong.

Occasionally, I have seen patients like Susan, a 45-year-old professional and mom who looks very healthy but has been suffering from migraine headaches, body pain, and breakouts of eczema for years. The chief complaint is almost always extreme fatigue. These patients eat right, exercise, don't drink, don't smoke, and their annual physicals find nothing wrong but they feel sick. Many times, these patients are placed on antidepressants.

These are difficult cases because most of them will have an exogenous cause. This means something from outside the body is disturbing or damaging their body. In these cases, the search for the exogenous cause becomes critical. First, we have to find and remove the outside source before we can normalize the system. In many cases, these patients have damage that may take some time to correct. Usually, we will find these patients have a food allergy, metal toxicity, or a disturbance in the nervous system. Often, they will have fungal infections associated with mercury or lead toxicity. Their Leaky Gut comes from damage from this exogenous source that is disrupting the transport system. These cases require significant workup and long-term digestive system treatment.

These warning symptoms are an indication that the active transport system is malfunctioning and breaking down. When the active transport system is working correctly, the materials and nutrients your body needs are escorted across the barrier, and all the things it doesn't want are left in the intestines to be pushed out of your body in the form of feces. If any part of what should end up as feces does leak across the lumen wall, you will get sick. The waste products belong outside of your body in the toilet, not in your bloodstream; it doesn't take much imagination to understand why you don't want waste products inside of your body. The active transport system of the digestive tract is the way your body keeps waste products in the intestines and takes the nutrients into the body.

CROSSING THE BARRIER WITHOUT AN ESCORT

Active transport uses energy (work) to move molecules that the cell needs, like glucose, amino acids, ions, minerals, vitamins, *when* they are needed and not before. It is the gate mechanism that protects the cell from unwanted and unprocessed materials and escorts the selected ones across the cell wall of the intestines into the bloodstream. This transport system is the key to health, and the breakdown of this system sets the stage for chronic illness.

The intestinal cell wall has a specialized barrier that protects it against unwanted substances, just like your skin protects you against the outside world. When this layer is damaged, unhealthy, overwhelmed, or attacked, unwanted substances can enter the cell without being escorted by the transporters. The body sounds the alarm through the nervous system that it has been invaded, and the immune system starts to wage a battle against these unwanted guests to eliminate them. The level of battle depends on the amount of damage to the cells and how much of the non-escorted substance gets into the body. A small battle may not produce many symptoms, but a war will usually cause sickness or severe symptoms that can be anything from migraines and chronic fatigue to serious autoimmune disease.

Any substance that the cell is trying to keep out is one of these unwanted guests, also known as antigens. The list of potential antigens is long and includes toxic chemicals such as mercury, aluminum, lead, cadmium, and a host of other heavy metals. It also includes chemicals that will injure the cell wall and disrupt hormones, which blocks and interferes with normal functions all over the body. Certain pesticides and chemicals, like food additives and preservatives, can act as disrupters. Other common antigens are bacteria, viruses, parasites, and waste products (i.e., anything that the body doesn't choose to have). But the most common antigen is undigested food particles that were not properly prepared and broken down earlier in the digestive process due to a lack of stomach acid, gastrin, and digestive enzymes.

When unescorted crossings of the lumen wall occur in the digestive tract, this is called Leaky Gut. Normally, the cells of the digestive tract barrier have tight junctions that ensure only escorted substances can cross. If there are holes or gaps between these cells, particles of all sorts are allowed to go directly into the bloodstream without an escort or transporter. Whether those particles are bacteria, virus, fungus, or chicken, the immune system will see it as an enemy and launch an attack. When the immune system attacks, inflammation occurs. When the digestive wall becomes inflamed, then the junctions open up due to swelling, allowing unwanted substances to cross the intestinal wall into the bloodstream without being selected and transported. A vicious cycle now develops. On top of this, toxic chemicals have the unique characteristic of being able to cross the barrier by moving right through the middle of a cell or hijacking a cell's receptors. Once they have forced their way through, they wreak havoc on hormonal systems and potentially any system of the body. For this reason, it is essential that potential antigens are eliminated by the stomach acid barrier before they make it into the small intestines.

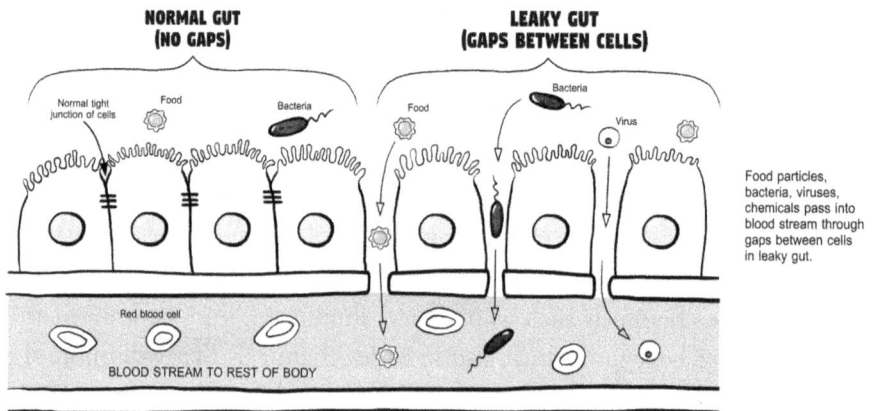

NORMAL GUT (NO GAPS)

LEAKY GUT (GAPS BETWEEN CELLS)

Normal tight junction of cells

Food

Bacteria

Food

Bacteria

Virus

Red blood cell

BLOOD STREAM TO REST OF BODY

Food particles, bacteria, viruses, chemicals pass into blood stream through gaps between cells in leaky gut.

The body's immune system is always on the lookout for these invaders and usually kills or destroys them very quickly. If your body is not breaking down food and escorting across the membranes in the small intestines with a properly operating active transport system day after day and week after week for years and years, your immune system is at continuous war. We see this on blood work with increased levels of two important immune markers—lymphocytes and neutrophils—and often with mildly elevated white blood cells. When your immune system is at war for decades against common foods that have not been properly digested, the result is fatigue, skin problems, autoimmune disease, sickness, and functional misery of life. The body eventually breaks down and chronic illness replaces health.

This process is the reason why "you are not what you eat"; rather, "you are what your digestive system determines you to be." When the gut has become leaky and substances are no longer being selectively escorted across the intestinal wall to the bloodstream through the active transport system, then any food, including nutritional supplements—no matter how "healthy" or "clean" it is—can cause problems because the system has become dysfunctional. While diet and nutrition are an extremely important aspect of health and healing, the first step must be repairing the Leaky Gut and restoring the digestive system to normal functioning. Otherwise, you are fighting a losing battle.

SYSTEM BREAKDOWN

The entire cycle of digestion begins with chewing the food, which breaks the substance down into smaller particles so the taste buds can analyze the chemicals. Through the nervous system, those chemicals communicate to the digestive organs what types of transporters are needed in order to process the food and deliver it into the cell through the membranes of the small intestines properly.

If just a few substances—like undigested food—breach the digestive wall, the immune system cleans this up pretty quickly. But if it happens over and over again for two weeks, the body's immune system starts to build an antibody to that antigen. Now, anytime these particles enter the bloodstream, the immune system will tag these particles and attack them as if they were dangerous bacteria or a virus. This "antigen-antibody complex" can cause a lot of problems, including chronic fatigue and autoimmune disease. It also often results in the development of a IgG antibody. The immune system produces several different types of immunoglobulins, or antibodies, that function to find the problem source and destroy it. IgE (immunoglobulin E) is the most well-known type of allergy antibody and results in the rapid reaction most of us are familiar with after being exposed to pollen, animal fur, or certain foods: runny nose, itchy eyes, sneezing, coughing, or even the throat closing up.

However, there are other types of allergies. Leaky Gut typically results primarily in an IgG allergy, which we measure with a blood test. The IgG allergy is a delayed reaction, from a few hours up to 72 hours after exposure, and results in different symptoms like fatigue, eczema, and migraines. The IgG allergy is what a functional medicine doctor is going to test. Most folks know about their IgE reactions because when they have been exposed to pollen or a food, they have had a reaction in the past. You can go for years and never know you have an IgG allergy because the body might take several days to react, which makes it challenging to identify. This is the result of the antigen-antibody complex. Substances that would normally be fine if properly digested instead leak across the gut wall into the bloodstream, signaling to the immune system that an invader has breached the wall and, with repeated exposure, causing the immune system to label that particular substance as a problem and setting the stage for delayed allergic reactions.

This reaction can manifest in many different symptoms depending on where the complex migrates to in the body via the bloodstream. During the immune system's process of attaching to and fighting the perceived invader at the site where it has migrated to, the immune system also has the capability of destroying whatever tissue it is attached to. When these complexes migrate and attach to the skin, it results in skin symptoms such as eczema or psoriasis. If this migratory complex migrates to the synovial fluid of the knee, the immune systems attacks it, which results in rheumatoid arthritis. If it attaches to the thyroid, it is Hashimoto's disease. If it migrates to the blood vessels of the brain, migraine headaches can develop. This is called autoimmune disease, because the body is attacking its own tissue. The fix for this is to stop the Leaky Gut.

Functional medicine doctors will sometimes test for IgA, which are antigens that are in the lining of the intestines. This test indicates if you are having a surface reaction in the gut that is of long-term significance. I don't test for these with simple cases of Leaky Gut. However, in complex cases or cases that don't respond as expected, IgA antibody testing is often appropriate.

When you understand this process, you can see that many of these autoimmune diseases and other conditions such as migraine headaches and eczema are really symptoms of a malfunction of normal function, not of a distinct disease entity. This is why there is no allopathic medical cure for these conditions. Allopathy only treats the symptoms because treating the "disease" itself will not solve the problem. The disease is the final result of many normal functions in the body not functioning normally.

To solve the problem, the root cause of the symptoms must be removed. Then, the "disease" resolves on its own because the reason for the eczema, headaches, or self-attacking of the immune system no longer exists. This is the basis for functional medicine. Find the breakdown of which system and correct it. With Leaky Gut, the substances are crossing the digestive tract membrane unescorted due to a disruption in the critical active transport process. This often starts because a lack of HCl in the stomach means that the food was not properly prepared for digestion, resulting in a cascade of downstream effects in the small intestine and beyond. Stomach acid levels are the first place to look and one of the first tests to run.

CHAPTER 6

Everything Is Connected

How Leaky Gut is interconnected with other essential bodily processes, and why they are important to address in treatment

Patients come to my office with a wide range of ailments and complaints, and they're often surprised that taking care of a problem in their digestive health can have such a dramatic impact on other parts of their bodies. And that's because it's all interconnected. Functional medicine understands and assumes that anything can cause anything.

AUTONOMIC NERVOUS SYSTEM

What people may not realize is that the nervous system (the brain, spinal cord, and network of nerves) is critical to the proper functioning of the digestive system. We cannot chew our food or even open our mouths without the nervous system working properly. Actually, we could not even get the food to our mouth without the nervous system that controls all of our movements, vision, and every aspect of bodily function as well as chemical reactions. While there are some aspects of the nervous system that we have control over, like the parts involved with picking up a fork, opening our mouth, and chewing, there are many aspects of the nervous system we have little conscious control over. This is the autonomic nervous system. It functions automatically without you having to think about it, like the lungs breathing, the heart beating, and the digestive tract processing food. This is the nervous system we are talking about when we discuss digestion and Leaky Gut.

When the taste buds analyze the chemicals in your food, that information is transported to the brain. The brain then decides what enzymes and chemicals need to be produced, what active transport machines need to be ready to go, how many are needed, and so on. Through a series of signals, the brain and individual cells throughout the body communicate with one another, starting the trillions of reactions that must take place to digest the food. All of this information allows the active transport system to identify what it doesn't want and keep the undesired substances "outside" the body in the lumen to be eliminated as waste. You don't have to think about any of this. It is done automatically.

An excellent example of the autonomic nervous system is swallowing food. After you make the decision to swallow the food, the autonomic nervous system takes over the process. The esophagus muscle uses alternating contractions to push the food down to the stomach. It takes about six seconds for the food to travel from the mouth to the valve on the top of the stomach, the valve to open up, and the muscles to push the food into your stomach. Now, if the valves fail to function properly, usually due to insufficient stomach acid levels, food can reflux back into the esophagus. If this happens, it can result in mid-back pain or chest pain and is oftentimes mistaken for a heart attack.

Since the autonomic system controls every function and goes to every cell, this means that every part of the body is connected to every other part of the body by the nervous system. Therefore, anything can cause anything because everything is connected to everything. Functional medicine has techniques to diagnose and treat the nervous system, and these systems must be addressed as part of the healing process.

PATIENT STORY: CHEST PAIN

Rick was experiencing intense chest pain. He was in his early 50s, so naturally he thought he was having a heart attack and went to the ER. The doctors ran their tests and told him everything was fine with his heart. Even though he was given a clean bill of health, he continued to have chest pains. Eventually, he found his way to my office. After we examined him and ran a series of tests, we found that his stomach acid levels were low.

While the connection between chest pain and digestion issues may not seem immediately apparent, it makes sense because of the way the nervous system functions. Nerves that connect the stomach to the nervous system originate from the middle of the back between the shoulder blades, and irritation in the stomach due to lack of stomach acid causes the muscle to spasm in that area. This can often present as back pain or chest pain and understandably leads some people to believe they are having a heart attack. In reality, it's often a digestion issue. In this case, the Gastro-Test® indicated hypochlorhydria. Rick was prescribed HCl and pepsin supplements along with enzymes, made minor changes to his diet, and all the chest pains stopped.

LIVER, GALLBLADDER, AND PANCREAS

The liver, gallbladder, and pancreas are our friends in digestion. The liver is almost never addressed in any discussion about gut health, yet it plays a significant and life-sustaining role in normal digestion. The liver is the major detoxification organ of the body, and it filters dangerous chemicals like arsenic, mercury, and lead. In simple terms, the liver breaks down toxic substances and makes them water soluble so they can be excreted from the body through the kidneys and bowels. Without the liver doing its job, these dangerous chemicals could be absorbed in the small intestine and potentially kill or harm us. Recently, it was discovered that the liver has cells that function in partnership with specialized cells of the small intestines called enterocytes. These cells in the small intestines function as "little livers," helping to filter and eliminate toxic metals, drugs, and unwanted chemicals. The fact that our bodies have a backup system to the liver in our small intestines indicates just how important the identification of dangerous chemicals is to our health. We don't think about our liver much, but it is so important that it is one of the first areas we address in functional medicine diagnosis and treatment.

The liver also performs one of the most important digestive functions in the body: it produces bile, which is critical for the digestion of fatty acids. After the liver produces bile, it collects and stores it in the gallbladder. The gallbladder squirts bile into the small intestines when fats need to be digested. Even though the word "fats" might sound like a four-letter word, it's important to understand that fats are not bad. In fact, they are essential and we would die without them. Fats contain fatty acids that make up the cell wall of every cell of your body. They are the key to slowing the aging process and to overall health. I tell my patients that, if I had only one nutrient to prescribe, I would prescribe the essential fatty acids. And that is actually what I do for every patient. If you have had your gallbladder removed, you need to supplement with bile salts at every meal for the rest of your life in order to avoid developing a fatty acid deficiency, of which the key symptoms are dry skin and hair.

The pancreas further assists with digesting fatty acids, as well as digesting carbohydrates and proteins, by producing digestive enzymes. The pancreas also produces insulin, which doesn't directly involve digestion but is very important at the cellular level to control blood sugar. Pancreatic enzymes include lipase, amylase, and trypsinogen. Lipase splits fats into fatty acids, amylase splits starch from carbohydrates to maltose (sugar), and trypsinogen splits protein into amino acids. Fatty acids from fats and amino acids from proteins are the building blocks of the body—from cells and hormones to bones and muscles—and sugar from carbohydrates is the fuel that provides energy for the body to function. If your body does not produce enough pancreatic enzymes, fats, proteins, and carbohydrates are not sufficiently broken down and your small intestine is unable to absorb all the nutrients you need in order to function. This can lead to a wide range of symptoms, including chronic fatigue, headaches, stomach pain, indigestion, skin conditions, and hormone problems. Remember, any symptom or condition can result from inadequate digestive function. Pancreatic enzyme deficiency is very common, which is why this is one of the tests I run with every patient in conjunction with stomach acid level tests, the Gastro-Test®, and other fact-finding examinations and tests.

LARGE INTESTINE

Measuring at about 16 feet long, the large intestine primarily works to absorb water and minerals such as salt from the substances that have been passed on by the small intestine. On average, the large intestine produces around three to four ounces of feces per day, of which about two-thirds is indigestible food and waste products and one-third is bacteria. Some of these bacteria synthesize vitamins like B12 and vitamin K, which are critical for maintaining healthy blood and nervous system functioning. These five pounds of bacteria are of extreme importance and are a major focus in treating Leaky Gut. In some cases, Leaky Gut is caused by an overgrowth or imbalance of these bacteria.

The large intestine is responsible for moving unwanted substances out of the body in the form of feces, which it does by pushing waste products along using the muscles that line the intestinal tract. Through the process of digestion, the stomach, small intestine, and large intestine stretch and trigger reflexes that move food and waste along in a process called *peristalsis*. This reflex is important, because it is connected to the nervous system and can become dormant if you are not moving your bowels regularly. Medical textbooks vary on how often you should have a bowel movement, but humans are designed to move their bowels every time they eat something. The reflex is triggered by the stomach stretching. Dogs have the same reflex, and they have to be trained to not have a bowel movement every time they eat. The minimum for good health for humans is to move your bowels once a day. In my clinical opinion and experience, if you do not have a bowel movement at least once a day, you are constipated.

Constipation is a serious symptom of digestive problems. If your large intestine is full of waste, there is no place for waste coming from the upper part of the digestive tract to go, and things start to back up in the system. This causes gas, bloating, reflux, serious overgrowth of bacteria, and sickness. Constipation is not normal. I have seen patients who don't have a bowel movement for a week or, in extreme cases, even up to a month. This is serious. In much the same way that the sewer pipes in your home would back up into your rooms if they were completely full, the same thing can happen in your body. In fact, it can get so bad that a condition called fecal impaction can occur, which requires medical intervention.

One of the most important treatments is to restore the reflex responsible for a mass movement of the large intestines, which expels the feces. This reflex is triggered by the colon expanding with feces and filling up the large intestines. If constipation is present with Leaky Gut, this large intestine reflex becomes dormant because the size of the colon remains past the firing point of this reflex. So, the first step in treating constipation is to remove the waste products, which allows the colon to return to its normal size, restores the reflex to its original function, and makes mass movements normal again. This takes several months to do.

Another key component of the digestive tract is the valve between the small and large intestines that keeps feces in the large intestine from entering the small intestine. If waste products were to be backed up into the small intestine, they would be absorbed in the body (and it doesn't take much imagination to grasp why this is bad). When this valve is malfunctioning, there is often pain in the low back just above the hip and in the lower right area of the abdomen. This valve is often treated in natural medicine with manual therapy that involves physically manipulating those areas back into alignment. Pain can also appear in the low back due to the fact that the large intestine is controlled by the nervous system and some of those nerves originate in the sacrum, the triangular bone between the hips at the bottom of the spine. The nerves originating from the sacrum control the colon and rectum, the final sections of the large intestine where digested food is processed and stored before exiting through the anus.

One of the most important functions of the large intestine is the absorption of water and minerals from the undigested waste. If a person has to have part of their large intestine removed due to a severe condition, such as colon cancer, and experiences regular diarrhea, they will undoubtedly have a deficiency of minerals and will experience dehydration. There is specialized testing that can be performed to identify these mineral deficiencies as well as testing to discover more about your colon health. The most basic stool test is the Indican test or Obermeyer's test, which is a simple in-office test that I always do in conjunction with pancreatic enzyme and stomach acid testing.

The large intestine is the first part of the digestive tract to treat, in my experience, especially if there is constipation. The five pounds of bacteria must be normalized and balanced, electrolytes must be restored, and the reflexes must be reconditioned so they are no longer dormant. Without a clean, normally functioning large intestine, there will be no healing of the stomach issues and no repairing of the Leaky Gut.

The Occult Blood Test is a simple, inexpensive tool to screen for particularly dangerous conditions that can occur in the large intestines, such as colon cancer, polyps, internal hemorrhoids, fissures, fistulas, and ulcerative colitis. Any blood in the stool on this test can be correlated with blood work and combined with other diagnostic techniques, such as scopes and imaging. I always include this test with patients to diagnose or rule out more significant health conditions.

***

KEY POINT SUMMARY

Before we discuss how to test for and repair Leaky Gut, let's review the most important things to understand about the digestive system.

1. **The key to health is a properly functioning digestive system.** Digestion begins with chewing, which serves to break down food so it is more easily digested and to analyze substances in order to send signals farther down the line about which chemicals, enzymes, and transporters will be necessary. Food then passes from the mouth down the esophagus to the stomach, which serves as a mixing tank. Once the food has been sufficiently broken down by hydrochloric acid, pepsin, and gastrin in the stomach, it passes to the small intestines for absorption. This area is the key to digestion and gut health, and dysfunction here results in Leaky Gut. The small intestine absorbs what is needed with the help of the liver, gallbladder, and pancreas, which assist with detoxification and breaking down fats, proteins, and carbo-hydrates into fatty and amino acids that are the body's building blocks and sugar that is the body's fuel. Whatever is not absorbed in the small intestine continues to the large intestine. Here, the waste continues to be processed, being moved along by muscles as water and minerals are absorbed until the remaining waste products exit the body through the anus in the form of feces. This entire process of digestion takes place inside the lumen, a tube that runs from the mouth to the anus, and is essentially the

outside world inside of the body, kept separate by the intestinal wall. The key to health is a properly functioning digestive system that breaks down, absorbs, and transports what the body needs and eliminates what is unneeded or harmful. Dysfunction in this system can result in a wide range of symptoms, ultimately leading to chronic illness if left untreated.

2. **Stomach acid plays an essential role.** Hydrochloric acid (HCl) forms the stomach acid barrier, which is essential for mixing and breaking down food in preparation for absorption in the small intestines. It is also critical for eliminating toxic and unwanted pathogens, such as parasites, bacteria, and viruses, that are trapped by mucus in the nose and mouth and subsequently swallowed. Without adequate amounts of acid in the stomach, insufficiently digested food and undesirable toxins and critters are passed along to the small intestines, setting the stage for dysbiosis and Leaky Gut. Stomach acid also controls pepsin, which is necessary for breaking down protein before entering the small intestine. On the one hand, too little stomach acid results in too little pepsin, which leads to improperly digested protein and causes a breakdown in the entire system. On the other hand, too much stomach acid is a red flag and signals the need for further medical investigation.

3. **In most cases, reflux is *not* caused by too much stomach acid.** Stomach acid levels are the key to opening the valve at the bottom of the stomach and keeping the valve at the top of the stomach closed. If you don't produce enough hydrochloric acid, the valves in your system will malfunction; the bottom valve will not open in a timely manner, meaning that the food is kept in the stomach to continue mixing and breaking down rather than being moved along to the small intestine. This causes the food to be pushed back up to the top of the stomach and the valve to leak into the esophagus, which results in symptoms like heartburn or even back pain. Reflux is caused by *too little* stomach acid, not too much stomach acid in most cases. Doctors typically treat reflux with

antacids because they were taught to do this in school and were not trained to test stomach acid levels. Antacids and acid-blocking drugs not only fail to address the root cause but also exacerbate problems by disrupting the normal digestive process.

4. **You are *not* what you eat.** Active transport across the microvilli (tiny hairlike structures along the intestinal wall that form a specialized border between the small intestine and bloodstream) is the heart of and the workhorse of digestion. This is where the transporters selectively escort the molecules of fat, protein, carbohydrates, minerals, vitamins, and essential substances across the protective barrier into the body via the bloodstream. If this border is breached (e.g., by food, pathogens, or toxic chemicals) or the active transport system is malfunctioning (e.g., inflammation has widened the junctions between cells), these molecules cross the border unaccompanied by their proper escort and enter the body. Whether it's a pathogen or an undigested food particle, the immune system identifies that as an antigen (non-self), or an enemy, and starts a war to protect itself. If this happens once, you likely would not even notice. If it happens repeatedly, even safe substances, such as certain foods you eat regularly, are tagged by the immune system and you develop a delayed allergic reaction to that substance. If this goes on three times a day, at each meal, 365 days a year, year after year, the war begins to take a toll on your health. Usually the first symptoms are gas, bloating, and constipation, then fatigue, and then everything from skin rashes and joint pain to depression and serious autoimmune disease. Fatigue is the most common symptom seen in patients with dysfunctional digestive systems. This Leaky Gut breach of the small intestine's specialized barrier is the most common cause. It's not true that "you are what you eat"; rather, you are what your digestive system determines you to be.

5. **Protein keeps the system running.** Digestive enzymes, carrier systems, and transporter molecules in active transport are made

from protein. In fact, every activity in your body, of which there are trillions, is run by protein machines. In order to function properly, you must absorb and metabolize protein. This depends on your digestion. If your digestive system doesn't work because it is not producing enough stomach acid to digest proteins, then you cannot make the machines necessary for the system to work. The entire body breaks down. It may be slow, but it is breaking down day by day.

6. **The nervous system is important to digestive health.** The digestive tract is controlled autonomically by your nervous system. In other words, digestion happens automatically, and you have no real conscious control over it except chewing, swallowing, and defecating, and even most of those processes are primarily autonomic. Moreover, constipation leads to the reflexes necessary for bowel movements becoming dormant, and the reflexes must be retrained and activated again through the nervous system. If you are not moving your bowels at least once a day, you have neurological problems in your digestive system that must be treated.

The Bottom Line: Health is all about the barrier in the digestive tract allowing in the right materials needed to build, repair, and run the body and keeping out the bad stuff. All of life—and more importantly, the quality of life—depends on how well your digestive system does its job.

CHAPTER 7

The Four Essential Tests

How four simple tests can change your health, and why the
Gastro-Test® is the missing link in functional medicine

There are four simple, inexpensive in-office or take-home tests that patients should insist on having their doctors run in order to assess any digestive issue or chronic illness:

1. Gastro-Test®

2. Indican Test

3. Occult Blood Stool Test

4. Pancreatic Enzymes Test

These four tests are the absolute minimum necessary to determine any level of Leaky Gut. Hopefully, at this point in the book, it is clear why symptoms are not diagnostic. Because our bodily systems are interconnected, anything can cause anything. Every disease and every dysfunction will share some of the same symptoms, whether that is fatigue, headaches, muscle aches, joint pain, swelling, redness, rashes, fever, numbness, or even mood changes. Instead of turning to Dr. Internet (which is one of the most dangerous activities for chronically ill patients), we need to instead turn to diagnostic testing to find out what is wrong.

THE MOST IMPORTANT TEST IN FUNCTIONAL MEDICINE

I learned about all of these tests during my advanced training in Diagnosis and Internal Disorders, with the exception of the most important one: the Gastro-Test®. Just like every doctor, I was taught that too much stomach acid was the cause of reflux and stomach problems. At some point, I came across what was called "the string test" at the time. I remember thinking what a great idea it was to test the stomach acid and actually see if there was too much or too little acid. So, I started using them. This simple test gave me the answer I was looking for to this foundational question: Does this patient have too much or not enough stomach acid? The answers changed the way I practiced, and this test became a critical tool in my healing tool kit.

Later, these tests disappeared and I could no longer purchase them. Unfortunately, there were no other comparable options for testing stomach acid. So, I hired a group of professionals and we redesigned and improved the test. In 2021, I finally received a patent on the Gastro-Test®. They are now available to health care practitioners worldwide through the Gastro-Test® company. However, many practitioners are unaware these tests exist and that there is a safe, simple, inexpensive in-office test to determine stomach acid levels. Every practitioner who practices functional medicine should be doing this test. It is the missing link in functional medicine.

I have performed thousands of Gastro-Tests® throughout my 30-plus-year career and have learned several key takeaways. The first thing I learned after introducing this test to my regular diagnostic evaluation was that 90% of patients do not produce enough stomach acid levels; this contradicts what we learn in medical training where it is assumed that patients have too much stomach acid. The second thing I learned was that correcting the low stomach acid was dose dependent, meaning that the amount of HCl supplement depends on the individual patient and is not a one-size-fits-all treatment. The third thing I learned is that correcting the stomach acid problem would often correct a lot of issues that seemed unrelated to stomach symptoms but were, in fact, part of the same underlying dysfunction: Leaky Gut.

Please know that no patient should ever take an acid-blocking drug or HCl supplement without taking this test first. It is essential that you know what your stomach acid levels are before starting any kind of treatment and that you work with a health practitioner who can knowledgably plan and support your treatment. Sadly, we have created an epidemic of stomach problems and chronic illness by prescribing acid-reducing drugs without testing stomach acid levels first.

GASTRO-TEST®

There are two stomach acid tests available to patients: the Gastro-Test® and the Heidelberg Test. While both are designed to measure stomach acid, there are significant differences between the two. I want to make the case for why I believe the Gastro-Test® is the best choice for patients.

The Heidelberg Test is a pill with a radio transmitter that, once swallowed, signals information to a receiver, which is interpreted electronically. It measures pH levels (or acidity levels) after any stomach acid has been neutralized with baking soda. Essentially, it measures the stomach's ability to react to an artificial neutralizing of HCl. The biggest reason why I don't use this test is because it doesn't measure the most important aspect of acid in the stomach: the stomach acid barrier. You may recall from earlier chapters that the stomach acid barrier is critical to health because of its role in eliminating dangerous pathogens and toxins before they reach the small intestines, leak across the intestinal wall, and cause the immune system to launch an attack. The stomach acid barrier can only be measured in a resting state. Rather than measuring the resting stomach acid levels, the Heidelberg only measures the stomach's response to a chemical suppression of acid.

The Gastro-Test® has several advantages over the Heidelberg. First, it measures stomach acid levels both at rest and after being naturally "challenged" (i.e., during the process of digestion). Both of these measures are essential to accurately diagnosing and treating Leaky Gut. Importantly, it does not use chemicals like baking soda or other chemicals introduced into the stomach. The second part of the test measures the ability of the stomach to respond and make adequate amounts of acid when challenged; this is done by naturally stimulating the stomach, not forcing it to respond to suppression. This gives us a thorough understanding of the stomach's state of health at rest and under a more natural challenge (i.e., simulating the eating of food).

The second major advantage of the Gastro-Test® is that your stomach acid levels are measured directly with your own stomach fluids. It is not an electronic computation of acid levels received by a radio beam in response to an acid-neutralizing chemical. Rather, it is a direct measurement of your stomach fluids, much like putting a drop of liquid on a litmus testing strip and observing whether it turns red (high acidity) or blue (low acidity). It is a simple but very powerful test that directly analyzes the current state of your stomach.

Last but not least is time and expense. The Heidelberg takes up to two hours in a doctor's office and typically costs between $500 and $1,000. The Gastro-Test® takes 10 to 20 minutes, the cost is usually less than $200, and results are ready in about 2 minutes. In some cases, the test can be administered at home.

The Gastro-Test® is deceptively simple. I like to tell folks that it is like a fork: it may be simple, but it is impossible to replace because it does a job that nothing else can do.

GASTRO-TEST®
The Stomach pH Company

In office medical device to measure stomach pH
See website for
instructional videos

In office use & results	No drugs required
Non surgical non invasive	No special equipment necessary

www.Gastro-Tests.com | info@gastro-tests.com
281.996.7701

INDICAN TEST

The Indican Test (sometimes referred to as the Obermeyer Urinary Indican Test) has been around for a long time. Essentially, it assesses the presence of harmful anaerobic bacteria that can cause bowel dysbiosis and Leaky Gut. As you might remember, dysbiosis is an intestinal condition caused by reduced levels of beneficial digestive bacteria in the small intestine, which leads to malabsorption syndrome. Bacterial overgrowth and drops in beneficial bacteria are one of the leading causes of Leaky Gut; the Indican Test measures both. It quantifies the level of *indoles* in the intestine by measuring Indican in the urine. Large amounts of Indican are a sign of high bacteria counts in the small intestines.

Overall, the test measures the extent of Leaky Gut Syndrome indicated by the breakdown of gut permeability and integrity caused by:

1. Diminished hydrochloric acid production

2. Diminished bile flow

3. Lack of digestive enzymes

4. Intestinal obstruction

5. Putrefaction of food in intestines (rotting of food in the intestines)

This simple test only requires a small amount of urine, is very inexpensive, and can be completed in about five minutes in your doctor's office. In combination with the Gastro-Test®, these are the simplest and most inexpensive sets of tests to determine and quantify Leaky Gut.

OCCULT BLOOD TEST

The Occult Blood Test is a take-home stool test that is simple to use and inexpensive. This is a necessary test to determine if something serious might be developing such as colon cancer, internal hemorrhoids, polyps, or ulcerative colitis.

Essentially, the test involves placing sheets of test paper into the toilet after a bowel movement and watching to see if the paper turns blue, which indicates a positive result. Don't be alarmed and spend all night on the internet if it is positive. There are many things your doctor has to consider with a positive test, such as diet, medical history, or even how much vitamin C you consume. Your doctor will discuss any positive finding with you.

PANCREATIC ENZYME TEST

Pancreatic enzymes (amylase and lipase) correlate highly with the Gastro-Test® and Indican Test. There are several ways to test the levels of pancreatic enzymes. I prefer blood samples for multiple reasons that are beyond the scope of this book. Your doctor may prefer something different. The key thing to know is that, when looking at these levels from a functional medicine lens, we use narrower ranges of scores (optimal, high normal, low normal) instead of the wide ranges you see below that are more typical in allopathic medicine.

Does it make sense that one person with pancreatic enzyme levels of 25 and another person with levels of 125 would both be considered "normal"? These are disease levels, not functional levels. In functional medicine, we would start with the mean of this range, which is 87. Normal would be 87 plus or minus about 20%, or 69 to 105. Ranges above or below this indicate dysfunction. Your doctor would have to compare this result to your other tests to determine if this needed to be treated.

Allopathic medicine rarely concerns itself with low numbers. Rather, they focus on high numbers because that could indicate a disease state or a serious condition that needs immediate attention. In functional medicine, we are concerned with levels that are too high and too low because we are looking to optimize health, not just treat disease.

TESTING BASICS

There are a couple of things I want to talk about when it comes to tests. First, they cost money, but without them it is impossible to make a proper diagnosis and adjust treatment. Second, many of the good tests will not be covered by insurance. The insurance company wants the doctor to make a working diagnosis of a disease and then run the test to see if they are right. This really is the wrong way to approach functional medicine; the proper way is to run the appropriate tests and examinations to discover what is wrong. This is the only way to practice functional medicine. Since that way isn't favorable for the insurance company, you often will have to pay for tests out of pocket.

Given how expensive testing can be, you might be thinking it will be a waste of money to order a bunch of tests when most of them will likely be negative. But a negative test is just as important as a positive one. This is especially true with something like a negative Occult Blood Stool, which allows you and your doctor to not be so concerned about serious diseases that might kill you. Negative tests put that concern to bed and let the doctor move on to other possible causes. Every negative test that rules out a serious disease process is a welcomed sight in a functional medicine practice.

Compared to 35 years ago when I started this type of practice, we have very advanced functional medicine testing today. These tests can measure just about anything you can afford to measure at a very sophisticated level, from bacteria and antibodies in the stool to DNA and everything in between. I use these more advanced tests when I get stuck or yield insufficient information from the simple testing. However, it is important to remember that the body is a self-regulating and self-healing machine, and we don't always have to dig down into every DNA strand to produce health and relief from pain and suffering. The simple tests often are enough to correct the primary causes of your problems. I generally recommend a common-sense approach that starts with simple and moves to more complex as needed.

I always start with the four gastrointestinal tests described above, blood work, and IgG allergy testing. Then I do a trial treatment program to see if the patient improves. If the diagnosis is correct and the treatment is appropriate, the patient should see improvement in symptoms within a few weeks. You may hear from some practitioners that "it took you a long time to get this way, and it will take a long time to improve." This isn't really appropriate in simple cases of Leaky Gut. You should not get worse before you get better. If you are not getting better within a week (and are following all the instructions), then the diagnosis isn't correct or the treatment isn't proper. Complications range from simple to very complex, but some of the more common ones are metal toxicity, neurological issues, and fungal infections, especially *Candida*. This is why your doctor is so important.

We have covered four simple tests that your doctor needs just to get started, but depending on your particular case, it may be appropriate to run many more tests. Your doctor has to know every one of these tests like the back of their hand. They have to know how to integrate these findings with your particular case and run everything through the 1,300 possible diseases that exist plus the thousands of physiological malfunctions that might be the root cause of your problems. This is not easy. It takes years of training and a lot of experience to put all this together. Your doctor had to graduate from a medical school of some sort (MD, DO, DC, ND), pass national boards, do an internship, then continue to study every day for years to learn all the things they were not taught in school. This is a daunting task, and most doctors are not willing to do this. With any luck, you can find one of these doctors in your area; if not, keep searching until you find one. We will explore the topic of what to look for in a doctor more in-depth in the final chapter.

FINAL THOUGHTS ON TESTING

Most successful functional medicine doctors will start with a very good history and physical exam and will have a core set of tests they want to run at the start. It might take a few visits to complete the exams and testing. Once all the results are in, they should share with you a report of findings, a diagnosis, and a treatment plan.

Please don't go on the internet and try to become your own doctor. And once you begin a program, don't order all kinds of supplements or start a new diet without your doctor's guidance. If you do any of these things, you are sabotaging yourself. Your doctor cannot make adjustments to your program if you are taking every new supplement or following every fad diet that is on the internet. They have a plan that incorporates massive amounts information with their training and experience. Be patient and trust the process.

CHAPTER 8

Healing and Repairing Leaky Gut

*How to treat the root causes of chronic illness, and why supplements,
proteins, fatty acids, and proper nutrition are essential to helping
the body heal itself*

Having a "Leaky Gut" means that there are functional problems with the cell wall itself, the same wall that is supposed to keep what's inside your digestive tract (the outside world) from leaking into the rest of your body. These gaps or microscopic holes in the wall of the cell allow substances to cross from the digestive tract to the bloodstream with no check system (active transport), which triggers your body's alarm (the immune system). Your intestinal wall should be like a solid wood front door, restricting anything from entering your home unless you open the door and allow the person to enter. If someone tries to break in, your home alarm system will sound appropriately. Leaky Gut is like replacing that solid door with a flimsy screen door. Many things can pass through it unrestricted, from small insects and dust to water and burglars, and your alarm will sound at each of these invaders because it cannot distinguish which of these intruders are real threats. Imagine how miserable it would be to live in a home with an alarm system that goes off in response to every little thing; this is effectively what is happening in your body when your gut is leaky.

In much the same way that the fix for this situation is to replace the screen door with a solid front door, the fix for Leaky Gut is to heal the gaps and microscopic holes in the tissue and replace them with a healthy lining that returns normal function of the tissue. How do you repair the cell wall of a Leaky Gut? It's a nutritional problem that has to be repaired with proteins, fatty acids, minerals, vitamins, and proper diet. When the cell wall is functioning properly, the body's intelligence knows what to let in and what to keep out based on the needs of each cell. The cells inside your body signal to the nervous system what they need to survive and be healthy. The nervous system processes that information and then signals to the transporters in the digestive tract what needs to be let across the intestinal wall and what needs to be kept inside the lumen. These transporters also must identify substances that are not prepared properly to enter the cell. If a piece of undigested food you have eaten is not properly broken down and prepared, it must be kept out of the cell or the immune system will target it as an enemy to be destroyed.

The body's intelligence determines what should enter and not enter. This happens automatically a trillion times each second without you knowing about it. What this means for you is that your body is designed to heal itself and capable of healing itself. In fact, this is the physician's greatest tool. Think about it for a second. If a doctor cleans and sews up a serious cut, all they are doing is approximating the tissue and cleaning it up to aid the process of the body healing itself. The same can be said for changing the chemistry of the body with nutritional or drug therapy. We are stopping the things that are injurious and adding the missing things to aid the body in directing itself back to health. This should be a great comfort to you to know that there is always hope. The natural state of a human is health, not disease and fatigue.

This repairing will occur naturally when Leaky Gut is treated properly. The process takes about one year at a minimum because there are millions of gaps and holes to repair. As you may have noticed, all of my patients' stories started with the same basic treatment: clean out the digestive system, address low stomach acid levels by supplementing HCl before meals, and correct deficient digestive enzymes. The dosages and length of treatment during this phase will depend on the patient's test results and individual response to treatment. Once the root causes of Leaky Gut are under control, then it is time to introduce the nutrients necessary to heal the tissue. The basic treatment consists of nutritional therapy with proteins, fatty acids, minerals, and vitamins along with proper diet.

THREE TREATMENT PHASES

Over the past several decades, I have developed and refined a three-phase treatment program that has proven effective at addressing the root causes of Leaky Gut, repairing the digestive system, and maintaining gut health long-term. While the specifics of the program are tailored for each individual patient, Leaky Gut treatment follows this general roadmap.

PHASE ONE: SYMPTOM RELIEF

The first thing to address is the lack of stomach acid if the Gastro-Test® indicates that HCl acid levels are too low, which is the case in at least 90% of patients. Often, patients also produce insufficient levels of pancreatic enzymes. So, the first treatment target is supplementing HCl before meals and pancreatic enzymes after meals. The second target is correcting dysbiosis, which involves a bowel cleanse. This corrects abnormal bacteria in the small intestines by killing and balancing abnormal bacteria growth and reducing fungal growth.

Testing plays an essential role throughout the first phase of treatment. The goal is to provide the minimal amount of treatment necessary to relieve symptoms by addressing the underlying cause, which is reflected in diagnostic test results. The Gastro-Test® and Indican Test are particularly important, and because they are so inexpensive and easy to carry out, we repeat these tests consistently to track our progress.

When symptoms have subsided and the patient has started to feel better, we then move on to the next phase.

PHASE TWO: HEALING

In the second phase, we turn our focus to healing the intestinal wall lining and replacing the flimsy screen door with a solid wood door. Our guts rely on two nutrients to function properly: amino acids and fatty acids. These building blocks of life come from our diet.

PHASE THREE: MAINTENANCE

The maintenance phase ensures that the gut does not become "leaky" again, which primarily involves avoiding the things that led to problems in the first place. While this can often be the most challenging phase of treatment, patients who commit to maintaining gut health enjoy energetic lives free from pain and other debilitating symptoms.

Over the years, I have learned not to do too much too soon. In the early days of my practice, I would start patients on supplements and nutritional programs at the very beginning; unfortunately, this sometimes made patients worse. While supplements and nutrition are essential to the healing and repairing process, the body must have a functioning digestive system, which means having adequate levels of stomach acid and pancreatic enzymes. The first phase lays the necessary groundwork for the healing and maintenance phases, where we focus on proper nutrition and supplements, particularly related to protein, fatty acids, vitamins, minerals, and nutraceuticals.

PROTEINS

I can usually tell when a patient is suffering from a chronic illness as soon as they walk into the office. When a person is healthy, there's an energy, a vitality, a shine in the eyes. In contrast, a person whose body is struggling has a slightly hunched posture, a strained smile, a dull sheen in their eyes and hair. Chronically ill patients always want to know, "How do I get back to my normal self? How do I find that spark, that energy again?" Part of the answer lies in how well proteins are digested, processed, and absorbed through the gut.

Proteins are formed from amino acids linked together by peptide bonds that fold into a peptide chain. These chains form into a specific shape, turning them into tiny machines that perform specific tasks in the cell such as carrying vitamins and minerals to different parts of the cell. They perform the trillions of tasks that must take place every moment in your body, from manufacturing neurotransmitters, which keep your nervous system running, to constructing DNA, the genetic blueprint that controls everything in your body. Protein is essential for life, and without it, body function breaks down and eventually leads to death.

In fact, I would argue that this protein issue is one of the keys to health. In every health problem, whether it is fatigue, body pain, or preparing for or recovering from surgery, the protein status is critical. Without properly digested and processed protein, you will not have health or freedom from disease. You will not heal from injury. You will not wake up every morning and look forward to living life to the fullest. If your doctor overlooks the fact that you have a protein assimilation issue and your body is not working properly at the cellular level, you and your doctor will be chasing your tails around and around for years. It makes no sense to tackle every virus, bacteria, toxin, and structural problem if the basic engine of every function of the body is broken down and not functioning properly. If the protein digesting system is broken down, the body cannot get well and you cannot obtain true health.

These miniature machines, the functional blocks of human life, are made of the protein you eat, broken down into amino acids. The body needs the best protein to make high-quality amino acid tools, and the digestive tract must perfectly process and absorb amino acids (or at least as near to perfect as possible). At this point in the book, hopefully it is clear how important stomach acid is to digesting and processing the right kinds of high-quality proteins. Just eating the best quality protein isn't the only answer. You must digest it and absorb it properly through the active transport in the digestive tract. All this starts with adequate levels of HCl in the stomach. If this processing is dysfunctional, these undigested proteins can become a source of all kinds of health problems.

Undigested amino acids that cross the intestinal barrier unaccompanied by active transport are treated by the body as non-self and are identified as "antigens" by the immune system. The immune system reacts to kill and eliminate these antigens even though they may have started out as a very high-quality protein such as organic chicken or beans. If this continues meal after meal and year after year, it can result in eczema, migraine headaches, fibromyalgia, body and joint pain, and autoimmune disease. **The number one cause of fatigue in my 30 years of functional medicine practice is Leaky Gut caused by lack of hydrochloric acid and enzymes that do not break down these amino acids properly in the stomach and small intestines.**

AMINO ACIDS AND DEPRESSION

Amino acids also impact mental health, particularly depression, because of their role in neurotransmitters, the chemical messengers made and released by the nerve cells that tell other cells what to do. A deficiency of certain neurotransmitters can cause depression, and protein is relevant because neurotransmitters are made from amino acids called "precursors." For example, you may have heard of a class of antidepressants called SSRIs (selective serotonin reuptake inhibitors), such as Prozac. These drugs presumably affect depression levels by decreasing the amount of serotonin that is broken down and reabsorbed, effectively increasing the amount of serotonin available to be used by the brain. The precursor to the neurotransmitter serotonin is an amino acid called tryptophan. Thus, levels of serotonin can be altered by taking the supplement tryptophan rather than taking an SSRI drug to interfere with the normal reabsorption process.

And here's the question every depressed patient who walks through my door asks me: "Why would amino acids be low in the first place?" The number one reason is hypochlorhydria, low stomach acid. To digest protein into amino acids for the body to use in producing neurotransmitters, the acid levels must be high enough to break them down in the stomach. If you have taken SSRI prescription drugs and it has helped, that is a good indication that neurotransmitters are the issue and testing for HCl levels is critical.

Feeling blue and unwell isn't necessarily depression. Being sick will make you feel "depressed." There are specific tests for amino acid deficiencies that can be performed after your digestive system has been addressed if your mood still has not improved. Amino acid therapy should be combined with a full functional medicine program to be effective. Remember also that one supplement like tryptophan is not the answer. Don't run off and take a bottle of tryptophan for depression. That is the allopathic approach of A for A and B for B. It doesn't work like that. Finding and correcting the underlying cause, starting with the digestive system, is the proper approach to depression, just like any other problem.

PATIENT STORY: DEPRESSION AND ANXIETY

John had a long history of depression and anxiety. He said he felt like his insides were vibrating, and he couldn't remember a time when he hadn't felt depressed and anxious. He had been treated for years with medications that he said didn't really help. He had even taken tryptophan and amino acids in the past with no results. Testing indicated that John's stomach acid levels were very low and his digestive system was not processing the proteins properly. When we addressed the low acid levels and functioning in the intestinal tract, he started absorbing the amino acid precursors for the neurotransmitters that I prescribed for his depression and anxiety. Within five weeks, his mood symptoms had resolved and haven't returned since. Bottom line: the first step in treating depression is a full workup and testing of the digestive system.

FATTY ACIDS

One of the main reasons for a chronic Leaky Gut is that the cell wall of the gut is made from the wrong fatty acids. Cell wall tissue is 90% fatty acids. These should be cis fats, not trans fats. Cis-fatty acids come from food sources such as avocados, nuts, olives, fish, and eggs. Trans-fatty acid foods are typically manufactured with a type of oil that makes the product more shelf stable; examples include fried foods, baked goods, and many processed foods.

The majority of the American diet is trans fats. If a child is raised eating the wrong fats over time, the surface of the gut barrier erodes and results in gaps and leaks. When the fatty acids or proteins are of inferior quality, the cell wall becomes defective. Often this begins at birth. Mother's milk is made primarily of fatty acids because every cell of the baby is primarily fatty acids. However, most formula is made from soy and cow's milk, which is primarily made up of protein and not fatty acids. If a child is raised on formula, they will not receive the necessary amount of fatty acids necessary to build the cell walls properly and will end up with a defective intestinal wall. Babies' intestinal tracts are not designed to digest all the protein in the formula. This protein leaks through the immature baby gut, the proteins in the formula become antigens, and the baby develops all kinds of problems, including chronic ear infections, eczema, gas, bloating, and colic. When I see these little guys with snotty noses, puffed-up eyes, and bloated tummies, I really feel sorry for them. The next step in allopathic care, after months of antibiotics, is usually tubes in the ears. Most of this can be avoided.

Even when mothers are breastfeeding their infants, sometimes Leaky Gut still occurs because of an issue with a food the mother is eating. When my daughter had her child, she made great efforts to be extremely careful with diet and lifestyle. She called me one day and said that her son, who was only on breast milk, was breaking out all over with red blotches. I told her it was something he was eating, and she said that was impossible since she was breastfeeding him. So, she came into my office and we tested her for food allergies. It turns out she was allergic to eggs and had been eating them daily. She stopped eating eggs, and three days later her baby's skin cleared up. As a doctor, she now helps many of her own patients who are breastfeeding.

The Gastro-Test® is still the right place to start to check for adequate levels of HCl in the stomach, though in these cases we would only perform the test on the mom, not the infant. Then, to treat this problem, changes in diet must be implemented and nutraceuticals containing the right fatty acids and protein along with other building materials must be taken as directed.

Another important function of fatty acids is weight management. Over the years, fats have earned a bad reputation, but the truth is that fats and proteins decrease hunger because they have what the body needs to function. When you eat proper fats and proteins, you naturally eat less and still feel satiated, which means you aren't loading up on carbohydrates. Ultimately, you should eat to produce health, not to lose weight. It is nearly impossible to be overweight if you are eating for health.

PATIENT STORY: WEIGHT LOSS

I was giving a speech years ago when a young woman who was about 35 years old stood up and asked me why she couldn't lose weight even though she had been on a fat-free diet for years. I told her to make an appointment at my office. When she came in, we tested her stomach acid levels and pancreatic enzymes, which were both deficient. After supplementing HCl and enzymes, I switched her to a diet with adequate fat and protein. She was very worried because she thought she would gain weight, so I explained to her she would not crave food because fats and proteins in the right amount would curb her hunger. She stuck with the nutritional program and lost 20 pounds over the next few months.

VITAMINS, MINERALS, AND NUTRACEUTICALS

Early in my career before I started testing stomach acid levels, I would often try to treat Leaky Gut with vitamins and minerals and commercially available Leaky Gut products. To my frustration, my patients got worse. Over time with more experience and advanced functional testing, I started to understand that it wasn't the product making them worse; it was the fact that, no matter how good the product was, if it wasn't processed and transported properly it became the antigen and the immune system attacked it. When I started testing the stomach acid levels and the other functional issues in the gut and addressed them first, I was then able to use these products effectively to heal the gut.

Over the years, companies developed a new type of supplement called nutraceuticals. They are researched, tested, and manufactured to very high standards and are much more than just minerals and vitamins. Nutraceuticals are naturally based products that are formulated to target a specific function in the body. I have found they can produce excellent results in the hands of qualified and experienced doctors who are trained in functional medicine.

NUTRITION

I will often tell patients at the beginning of their program that when they finish going through the produce and meat section at the grocery store to just go straight to the checkout. That might sound harsh, but when your gut is sick, you should not eat processed foods like protein drinks and boxed or canned foods. They are too concentrated. Treat these processed foods as potential antigens until we can heal your gut. Be patient. When you get well, you will be able to tolerate some of these foods. Until the digestive system is functioning properly, focus on eating whole foods that must be chewed. Number one priority is making sure you are digesting proteins and fatty acids. We get both protein and fatty acids from the food we eat. The best source of protein is meat, which has all nine essential amino acids, meaning your body cannot make them from other materials so you must get them through food. In my book, if it flies, swims, or walks, it's meat. If you are on a vegetarian diet, you will need to supplement with medical-grade amino acid supplements, along with B12 and folic acid. It is very difficult to be on a pure vegetarian diet and get all the essential amino acids and fatty acids necessary for life.

Another important consideration with nutrition is rotating foods. You might recall from an earlier chapter that even undigested food particles can cross the intestinal wall unescorted, triggering the immune responses. If this happens over and over again for approximately two weeks, your body starts to develop an allergic reaction to it. So, I recommend that my patients rotate foods every other day, particularly protein types. Fruits and vegetables usually don't have to be rotated, but it is a good idea to do so in the very beginning of treatment. Also, in the first two weeks of most cases of Leaky Gut and dysbiosis, complex carbohydrates like rice, potatoes, and breads should be limited. These carbohydrates inhibit the balancing of the natural bacteria in the intestines. Additionally, allergy testing (IgE, IgG, IgA) is a helpful starting point for identifying foods you might be allergic to and need to avoid entirely.

HEALTH AND HEALING

We humans are made of dirt; it may be pretty sophisticated dirt, but it is dirt nonetheless. What this means is that we are highly adaptable and capable of change. Why would that be? Well, it is much easier to change a bunch of loose organic chemicals to adapt to some new environment than to change something rigid like titanium. **The body has the capacity to heal itself if we supply it with quality proteins and fatty acids, and we ensure that the digestive system processes and absorbs those substances**

in a functional way. The body can adapt at the cellular level just like we can adapt in our life. If it is cold, we can put on a coat. However, there are limits. If the weather is too harsh, no number of coats will prevent us from freezing to death. Our cells face the same strengths and limitations. They can be poisoned with waste products, damaged, starved to death, and become unhealthy because they are not supplied with the amino acids from proteins to maintain the cell. They will adapt until they can't change anymore. They either produce illness at that point, or they die.

Health is the ability of our body's cells to adapt to their environment. We call this cellular environment the *cellular matrix*. This is the living quarters of our cells. The health of that matrix determines what the cell is going to do and how it will adapt. If a matrix has no toxic chemicals, all the vitamins, minerals, water, etc. it needs, and all the right amounts and types of amino acids accompanied by their escorts, the cell functions normally and it is healthy. However, if any of those factors are not normal, the cell must adapt to survive. It has a tremendous ability to change and adapt to survive and will do everything it can to function. When it cannot function normally because of the abnormal cellular environment, then it changes its function to survive. That change is often the source of sickness and disease.

If an environmental change is small, we may only see minor problems like aches and pains. But large changes can produce serious disease and even death. At some point, the system breaks down and you start experiencing symptoms like rashes, stomach problems, body pains, or headaches. Remember, these are the symptoms, not the real problem. The worse the symptoms are, the more loudly your body is trying to tell you something is wrong. These symptoms are not an antidepressant or pain reliever deficiency. They are warning signs to you that your body is in trouble. Pain, in particular, is a sign that your body needs help.

Pain is produced when some group of cells is dying or seriously injured. Generally, there are two types of pain: sharp and dull. Sharp pains, like stabbing muscle or joint pain and migraines, are produced when these cells split open and the insides of the cell enter the cellular matrix and touch the nerves that monitor those cells. Dull pains, like the achy feeling you get with the flu and bloating, are produced by excess water surrounding the cells, which creates higher levels of hydraulic pressure. Both types of pain are innate alarm mechanisms; the cells trigger pain so you will know something is wrong, broken, sick, or damaged. Pain means you have cells that cannot adapt anymore and they want help. **Never ignore pain. It is the fire alarm of the body.** It means cells are being injured or destroyed and are in trouble. Drugs may help dampen the fire alarm, but in order to address the root cause and put out the fire, you need to get your digestive system functioning properly again, starting with adequate levels of HCl, and supply your body with high-quality proteins and fats.

IMPORTANT NOTE ABOUT GETTING BETTER

For the chronically ill who start to feel normal, it can be both an exciting and scary experience because you start to worry that feeling better will be short-lived. This is why functional diagnosis is so critical for the chronically ill: it helps you understand what dysfunction is causing your symptoms and what root causes you need to address in order to help your body naturally heal itself. When you make changes that produce health, you cannot go back to eating or doing the things that made you sick or you will get sick again. The idea that a magic drug will cure you is a great marketing ploy the allopathic medical community has sold to the public for centuries, but it is a false promise. If you stop doing the things that are making you sick and do the things necessary to produce health, you will feel better. It really is that simple. If you commit to making those changes, you don't have to worry about chronic illness returning and can look forward to a long life of good health. The first step is to find a doctor of chiropractic, licensed naturopath, osteopath, or medical doctor who has been trained in functional medicine and who can guide you through this process.

The information presented in this chapter is far from comprehensive and is not intended to be a guide for patients to create their own treatment plan. Rather, I hope to give you a broad sense of what effective treatment can look like and offer you the tools and terminology to make informed decisions about your own care. At this point, you have a solid grasp of what Leaky Gut is, why hydrochloric acid in the stomach plays a vital and often overlooked role in digestive functioning, and how to start the journey towards health and vitality. When you go to your health care provider, ask them what they think about Leaky Gut or dysbiosis and learn more about their approach to medicine and their diagnostic testing process. You need someone who is familiar with these ideas and takes them seriously, or who is at least willing to learn more about the topic and support you in carrying out basic diagnostic testing including the Gastro-Test®. Keep searching until you find the right health care provider for you.

CHAPTER 9

Finding the Right Provider for You

*How to navigate the process of finding a health care provider
who can help you, and why functional medicine offers hope to the
chronically ill*

Over the decades, I have become gentler and more conservative in my treatment of the chronically ill patient. We spend more time on diagnosing and finding dysfunction before coming to conclusions about treatment options. Because the body is a self-regulating and self-healing organism, it makes sense to start with the basics.

In the thousands of cases I have treated, a simple bowel cleanse program and normalizing stomach acid levels are often enough to solve very big problems within a few weeks, especially skin problems, eczema, headaches, and fibromyalgia. There is no need to run thousands of dollars' worth of tests and go on a restricted lifestyle that is barely livable. Sometimes, though, I run into the extremely complex cases such as metal toxicity causing neurological problems like seizures and tremors or the more serious diseases such as Parkinson's or multiple sclerosis. These complex conditions require a complex approach. The basic bowel cleanse and normalizing abnormal function of the digestive system are still the right place to start, but these patients will require more testing and investigating and their treatment will take longer.

Regardless of whether you are one of the 80% whose symptoms will resolve with a simple approach or one of the 20% who will have a more complex case, you need a health care provider, or a team of providers, whom you can rely on and trust to guide you through the healing process.

With the goal of helping you find the right kind of care, I want to share with you an overview of what kinds of providers are out there and how to determine if they could be the right one for you. In general, I recommend working with a provider who: (1) earned their degree from an accredited institution and is licensed by a state board, (2) has post-graduate training in functional medicine, and (3) has a reputation for being a good clinician.

FUNCTIONAL MEDICINE

Earlier in the book, we explored the differences between allopathic (conventional) and functional medicine. This is an important distinction to understand, as this is at least somewhat correlated with the type of medicine they studied and the type of license they have. If we think of providers as detectives following the clues, allopathic doctors would best be understood as "disease detectives," and functional medicine practitioners would be "physiological detectives." In other words, one is looking for clues that lead to disease and the surgical or pharmaceutical intervention that will cure that disease, while the other is looking for clues about dysfunctional processes and how to support the body in healing itself. While the allopathic approach focuses on diagnosing diseases and treating symptoms, the functional approach centers on identifying dysfunction and restoring health to underlying bodily processes.

Successful functional medicine practitioners generally fall into one of three categories. One is the individual who became sick themselves and found functional medicine through the process of answering all the same questions you are faced with. They ask themselves: "Where do I go to get help because what I learned in school doesn't work for my problem?" Another category is the curious, bright individual who is disappointed to learn that what they were taught in school doesn't allow them to heal patients. They start looking for other options to do what is right for patients and eventually find their way to functional medicine. Lastly, there is the scam artist. Yes, there are plenty of crooked doctors who will take you to the cleaners. These doctors get into functional medicine for the money. You may have seen clinics where you can walk in for a vitamin IV treatment and where a medical director is nowhere to be found. This is not functional medicine; it is a money machine. However, depending on resources available in your area, you might have to use one of these clinics under the direction of your doctor. Leave no stone unturned when it comes to where and how to get the help you need.

There are hundreds of doctors advertising they are functional medicine experts. Be careful. In addition to checking their accreditation and licensure, one of the best ways to determine whether someone is a real functional medicine provider is that they do their own history and physical. No physician—whether a DC, ND, DO, or MD—can be a top-notch functional medicine practitioner unless they personally take your history and perform your physical exam. If you go to a provider who does not take a history by sitting down and speaking with you about your issues, you are in the wrong place.

TYPES OF MEDICAL PROVIDERS

While we tend to use the term "doctor" to describe health care providers, there are actually a number of types of practitioners who can practice functional medicine and do not have "MD" after their names. The most common ones include Doctors of Chiropractic Medicine (DC), Doctors of Osteopathic Medicine (DO), Doctors of Naturopathic Medicine (ND), and Nurse Practitioners (NP). Each field has its own licensing board, so make sure that any provider you are working with is board certified in your state. Also, keep in mind that everyone in a particular field has to pass the same rigorous exams to earn their degree and license, so the "prestige" of the school they attended does not carry the same weight as it does in academia. Is a doctor who graduated from Harvard Medical School an inherently better functional medicine practitioner than a doctor who graduated from Podunk Medical School in Backwoods, Idaho? No; they took the same test to obtain a license. Moreover, functional medicine is not taught in medical school of any type and can only be learned in specialized training experiences. So, when selecting a physician to help you, pay attention to their post-graduate training because that will give you much more useful information about their background and expertise.

CHIROPRACTIC PHYSICIANS (DC)

Chiropractic Physicians are licensed in all 50 states, and there are Boards of Examiners in every state. The key to finding the right chiropractic doctor is to search out their post-graduate education and certifications. For example, I am a Board-Certified Chiropractic Internist with a Diplomate from the America Board of Chiropractic Internist and a Board-Certified Advanced Practice Chiropractic Physician. I am also certified in acupuncture, nutrition, neurotherapy, IV therapy, and a half-dozen other things. I have certificates for all of these, and the major specialties are recognized by the Board of Examiners in every state. All of these degrees are from accredited schools. These certificates are hard to achieve, which is why doctors are proud to display them on their walls.

My education and training are not necessarily the same as the chiropractor down the street treating neck and back pain. Chiropractic is like dentistry in that way. Any dentist can extract a wisdom tooth, but a board-certified oral surgeon has significant additional training in surgery. However, if a regular dentist has the right training and certifications, they are equally qualified to perform the same services as an oral surgeon. The same is true in the chiropractic doctor's case; chiropractors are all trained to treat neck and back pain (among other things), but chiropractors who also practice functional medicine must have additional certification. So, make sure your chiropractic physician has formal advanced training in functional medicine in post-graduate work.

One of the most advanced functional medicine trainings in our field is the Diplomate in Diagnosis and Internal Disorder (DABCI). This chiropractic physician has been trained in functional medicine and has passed rigorous tests required by the National Board of Chiropractic Examiners. While looking for a practitioner with this certification is a good place to start, there are many fine chiropractors who are excellent functional medicine doctors but don't have this specialty. Do your homework. There are great chiropractic doctors out there, just not on every corner.

NATUROPATHIC DOCTORS (ND)

Naturopathic Doctors are not licensed in all 50 states. There are several schools around the country that are accredited but many more that are not. If your state licenses NDs, there will be a Board of Naturopathic Examiners and they will allow only doctors who graduate from an accredited school to be licensed. Many NDs will advertise that they are certified. This is not the same as being licensed. The accredited schools are legitimate schools of naturopathic medicine, and their doctors are well trained in functional medicine concepts. These doctors will have a license in a state where licensing of naturopathic doctors is legal.

You will also sometimes see licensed doctors such as DCs, MDs, or DOs who advertise an ND degree in addition to their licensed degree. If that doctor is licensed in their primary training in your state, the additional ND or NMD indicates that the doctor has some training in naturopathic medicine. Some states, like Texas, will not allow doctors to advertise any degree they do not have a license for; since NDs are not licensed in Texas, most advertised NDs did not graduate from an accredited naturopathic college. Most states do not license NDs, so be careful. Find out if your state has a Board of Naturopathic Examiners and see if that practitioner is licensed.

MEDICAL AND OSTEOPATHIC DOCTORS (MD, DO)

While DOs historically practiced something closer to natural medicine, today there are very few differences between MDs and DOs. The training and testing is almost exactly the same, and they are considered full allopathic physicians by most insurance companies, the military, and the government. Both are highly trained and are experts in drug therapy and surgery. Having been thoroughly trained in disease care, it is extremely difficult for either of these types of doctors to convert to functional medicine. They do not share the same thinking process as functional doctors; diagnosing physiological dysfunction is just a fundamentally different way of thinking.

My observation over the years has been that it is more difficult for a DO or MD to practice functional medicine than a chiropractic or naturopathic doctor to incorporate allopathy into their thinking. Most DO and MD doctors I have seen who are involved in "functional medicine" still have an allopathy type of practice where they look for a disease; instead of treating the disease with standard drugs, they treat with a natural substance like herbs or homeopathy. This approach may work for some issues, but very few chronic diseases will be "cured" with this type of treatment. However, the DO and MD are the only ones who have total freedom to use any treatment they choose, so you may have to find one of these doctors to receive a treatment not available from chiropractic physicians or naturopathic doctors.

I tell my patients to keep their relationship with their MD or DO if they have a good one, because they will need their prescription pad, invasive testing, or surgical skills one day. The MD and DO have a monopoly in health care, whether we like it or not. So, try to find the best one you can.

NURSE PRACTITIONERS (NP)

In recent years, nurse practitioners have become primary care providers for allopathic medicine under this new corporate model of medicine. Like MDs and DOs, NPs are only trained in allopathic medicine. In most states, they work under an MD/DO supervisor who determines how they practice. However, in some states, nurse practitioners have the freedom to be "unsupervised," and in some cases these nurses have expanded into functional medicine. Some do procedures, such as pelvic exams and injections, that you might need and that may not be available from the functional medicine physician you are working with. In my experience, I have found in most cases nurse practitioners interested in functional medicine are very bright and open to working with the DC or ND, which is not the case with the majority of the MD/DO practitioners.

EXPECTING THE IMPOSSIBLE

Given the differences in training, it is important to manage your expectations. Don't expect an MD or DO to understand chiropractic or naturopathy or physiological medicine, and don't expect a chiropractic physician to endorse the use of drugs, surgery, or disease care approaches. Learn to use each appropriately; depending on the severity of a case, patients may need to work with a variety of medical providers.

The DC, ND, MD, and DO spend a minimum of 8 years of university and professional study just to become a doctor and another 10 years learning their craft either in the labs, hospitals, or clinics. It is silly to think anyone who spends decades learning one way of thinking is going to truly understand the other discipline's way of thinking. You wouldn't expect to buy a Ford at a Chevrolet dealership. Don't expect any doctor to abandon their decades of thinking and training a certain way for the unknown.

On top of the ingrained thinking, the emotional element makes it even more impossible. I once received a call from an MD who was getting started in homeopathy. He was scared to death he would hurt someone with a homeopathic medicine. I had to chuckle at the thought that it would be scarier to use a medicine that the FDA says is nothing but water than to use FDA-approved drugs that kill and injure patients regularly. He was emotionally uncomfortable with the homeopathy but comfortable with the prescription drugs. Chiropractic physicians and naturopathic physicians are just the opposite; they are emotionally uncomfortable with the prescription drugs. After years of training in this way of thinking, the only possibility is for each to academically understand the other side, even though they will never agree with it in their heart of hearts.

When you understand this, you can use each kind of doctor appropriately to solve your problems. I have a drug license but 99.9% of chiropractic physicians don't. Even with my training and drug license, I rarely prescribe a dangerous drug. My thinking is to try to avoid them because they don't heal. MDs and DOs view the role of drugs differently; their philosophy is drugs first and natural remedies later. In fact, some states mandate that allopathic doctors use drugs and surgery first and do not allow the use of safe medicines such as herbs until the dangerous drugs or surgeries fail.

So, how do you balance working with doctors from different backgrounds with different perspectives? First, all health care providers should understand their role in your treatment. If a doctor is hostile to you because you are seeing another provider, discuss it with them. You need both doctors even if they don't understand one another. I have seen many medical doctors refuse to treat a patient of mine because they see a chiropractor. This is blatant disrespect for the patient. If this happens to you, it is time to replace that doctor. Ultimately, you are the one who suffers, so it's important to learn to work with both sides of the fence.

FAMILY RELATIONSHIPS

Do you ever wonder what happened to the family doctor, the physician who lived down the street and treated your whole family?

Years ago, my son came home from surfing with a nasty cut on his foot. It wasn't bad enough to go spend all day in the emergency room, but he needed a couple of stiches. I called every family medicine clinic in the area, and they all referred me to the emergency room. Finally, I found someone halfway across town who put a couple of stiches in my kid's foot.

Medicine has become so specialized in dividing up the body that we have lost touch with the most important part of being a doctor: building relationships with patients and their families. Medicine is not just running tests and trying to find the next disease to treat. Primary care has been delegated to nurses and physician's assistants in corporate medical offices. This is one of the major reasons why the general public is becoming so dissatisfied with medicine. Families need a trusting relationship with a primary care doctor who knows them well and can help guide them through the system.

When I have a child come into the clinic and the parent(s) is also one of my patients, I have a huge advantage in figuring out what the problem is for the child. I know the health of the parents and I know a bit about their lifestyle, such as where they live, what they do for fun, and what they eat and drink. I know if they will follow directions and if they are serious about their health or if they are looking for a "miracle quick fix." In short, I am part of their family. If I have built a level of trust with this family, they know they can confide in me. This information might be the difference between life and death, either for themselves or someone they love. This relationship with your doctor is absolutely necessary to produce health.

Allopathic medicine, however, has decided that it is an industry and that corporate medicine is better than individual doctors with independent clinics. I think this is a huge mistake for our society. Human beings are not machines, and a singular system of industrial medicine will not work treating them as such. When you are looking for a doctor who is a healer, he or she will in all likelihood work independently, not for a medical group. They may have small offices that are not fancy. They will often be chiropractic physicians and not medical doctors or osteopaths. In some states, they are licensed naturopathic doctors.

FINAL THOUGHTS

If you take away one message from this chapter, let it be this: *do not try to do this on your own*. It takes many years to make a good functional medicine physician. Even the worst of them is better than Dr. Internet. Be smart and get help from a legitimately degreed and licensed professional.

I am an old warhorse who has been in the field for over three decades. I struggle to keep up with the latest basic sciences because I spent 30 years going from room to room helping patients. I study in my spare time and do my best to follow the latest developments. But there are plenty of old tried-and-true treatments that are as good as gold. New isn't always best. Wisdom and experience are worth much to you and your health

When I graduated from Louisiana State University a long time ago, I went into the U.S. Army and attended Army Flight School. It was the toughest thing I have ever done in my life. If we didn't learn to do everything in the right way and didn't perform to a certain standard, we knew that we were going to die in a smoldering pile of burning magnesium and aluminum. Not only would we kill ourselves but we would also kill everyone with us on our aircraft. It taught me responsibility and instilled in me how important procedures are in life.

As doctors, we deal with a different kind of pressure; rather than running the risk of getting ourselves killed if we don't do our job well, it is your life in our hands. I used to tell students who would come to the clinic that it is one thing to know the answer on the test; it's another thing when a human being sits in front of you and tells you, "I don't feel well. I have been to every doctor on my insurance. I need help. Please help me." That is the moment of truth for a doctor. If your doctor doesn't care, fails to understand their responsibility, or is unwilling to do the right thing for you as the chronically ill patient, then you are in the wrong place.

How do you know if they care? The first thing is simple: Do they take a good history, perform a complete physical examination, and tell you exactly what they are going to do? It isn't the personality. Who cares if the pilot flying the airplane is a great guy? Isn't the important thing that he is competent at flying airplanes? The same is true with your functional medicine doctor. Even if they don't have shining personalities, they may very well be great doctors. Judge them by what they do, starting with the history and physical. I cannot tell you how many thousands of patients were shocked that I look in their ears, listen to their hearts and lungs, and check their abdomen. Your doctor's actions tell you who they are, not their personality.

Functional medicine doctors are made after school, so don't expect one three weeks out of school to be a wizard. They may be learning and should not be ruled out just because they are new. If they are still studying, they may have learned exactly what you need last week in their post-graduate classes. In my earlier days, I used to tell my patients, "I'm learning everyday so if I don't know now, I might know soon. I promise I will never give up on you." I cannot tell you how many patients returned a few years later to find out what I couldn't fix then was an easy fix today.

With the help of a doctor who leaves no stone unturned, you will find relief from the symptoms that are holding you back. Don't lose hope. Remember: there is always an answer.

Gastro-Test®

Why guess when you can test?

If you are a patient struggling with chronic fatigue, pain, digestive issues, or other mysterious symptoms, ask your functional medicine provider to visit our website or contact us by email or phone to learn more about the Gastro-Test®. More than likely, your provider is not aware that it even exists. Most functional medicine doctors will be excited about a test that is so simple, inexpensive, and easy to do and that will give them a clear answer to a question that is foundational to health.

Our team is available to help practitioners order and perform the test and interpret results. If you cannot find a practitioner who will administer the test in your area, contact us and we will assist you.

GASTRO-TEST®
The Stomach pH Company

In office medical device to measure stomach pH

See website for
instructional videos

In office use & results	No drugs required
Non surgical non invasive	No special equipment necessary

www.Gastro-Tests.com | info@gastro-tests.com
281.996.7701

Epilogue

A NOTE TO HEALTH CARE PROVIDERS

If you are a practitioner of functional medicine, you understand how important digestion is to health. If digestion is impaired, good health is impossible. You now have a new tool in your toolbox. The Gastro-Test® will tell you unequivocally the most important starting point in gastrointestinal health. You no longer have to assume that too much acid is the problem or that every patient needs hydrochloric acid. In fact, either approach is bad medicine. It is especially dangerous to prescribe acid blockers to a patient who is already hypochlorhydric. In this case, you would be driving that patient into sickness and disease instead of healing them. Atrophic gastritis that is drug induced is not something most functional medicine doctors or practitioners want on their conscience.

Do the test. It is inexpensive, simple to use in your office, and gives you objective findings to base your treatment on. It is the missing link in functional medicine.

Visit www.Gastro-Tests.com to get started with testing your patients. If you have any questions about administering the test, interpreting results, or treating hypochlorhydria, you can contact us by phone or email (contact information is listed on the website).